electrocardiography

HENRY J. L. MARRIOTT, M.D., F.A.C.P., F.A.C.C.

Director of Clinical Research, Rogers Heart Foundation, St. Petersburg, Florida; Director of Coronary Care Center and Director of Electrocardiograph Department, St. Anthony's Hospital, St. Petersburg, Florida; Clinical Professor of Medicine (Cardiology), Emory University School of Medicine, Atlanta, Georgia; Clinical Professor of Pediatrics (Cardiology), University of Florida, Gainesville, Florida.

The Williams & Wilkins Co. *Baltimore*

First Edition, February, 1954
    Reprinted 1954
    Reprinted February, 1956

Second Edition, August, 1957
    Reprinted April, 1958
    Reprinted June, 1961

Third Edition, June, 1962
    Reprinted May, 1964
    Reprinted January, 1965
    Reprinted December, 1966

Fourth Edition, May, 1968
    Reprinted July, 1968
    Reprinted June, 1969
    Reprinted March, 1970
    Reprinted August, 1971

Fifth Edition, May, 1972
    Reprinted February, 1974

Library of Congress Catalog Card Number 78–185965 SBN 683–05572–0

composed and printed at the
Waverly Press, Inc.
Mt. Royal & Guilford Aves.
Baltimore, Md. 21202

practical electrocardiography

FIFTH EDITION

"For he who'd make his fellow-creatures wise
Should always gild the philosophic pill."

W. S. GILBERT

practical

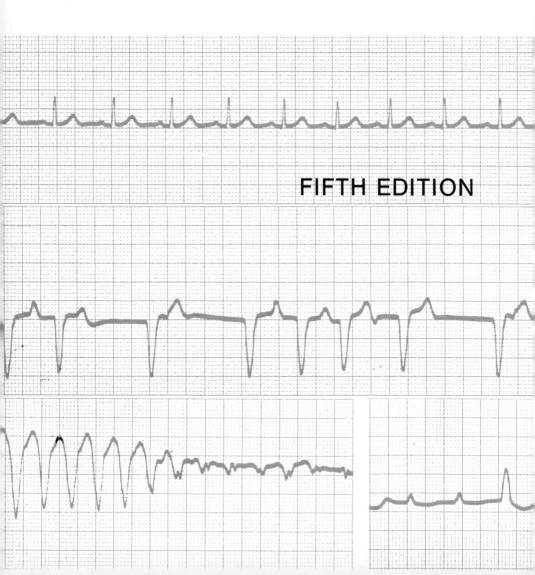

FIFTH EDITION

TO
Gladys

—who came back!

Preface to Fifth Edition

At about the time the first edition of this book appeared, electrocardiography as a subject for profitable progress and investigation was widely regarded as "dead." The events of the ensuing 18 years indicate that this assigned moribund status represented a gross misjudgment.

Since the last edition alone, numerous facts have emerged concerning the important differentiation of ventricular aberration from ectopy; new evidence has added to our confusion about the localizing value of P-wave patterns; new theories and facts have appeared which influence our concepts of the Wolff-Parkinson-White syndrome; His-bundle recordings have provided electrocardiographers with a fascinating new research tool and have confirmed many tenets hitherto precariously poised on postulates derived from clinical tracings; monitoring of arrhythmias and blocks in coronary care has achieved greater precision; and the whole subject of the hemiblocks has surfaced.

All these subjects have, therefore, been introduced or revised in the present edition. In addition, sixty new figures have been added as well as numerous key references, chosen with an eye not only to their value but also to their accessibility.

After each of the last twelve chapters, review tracings without descriptive legends have been inserted to serve as a cursory refresher course and as a stimulus to master what has gone before.

Aphorisms have always been helpful in teaching and learning because, as Osler picturesquely put it, they are "burrs that stick in the memory." I have therefore inserted at strategic points in the text several homespun epigrams that have seemed helpful, and these are appropriately tagged with **.

The aims and scope of this book are unchanged and simplicity remains the central theme. The text is designed to be digestible for beginners, yet not without value to those who already have a nodding acquaintance with electrocardiography. Once again the publishers have graciously given me a free and unconventional hand in arranging the layout of pages so that I have been able to place illustrations and descriptive text in as convenient proximity as possible.

H. J. L. M.

Preface to First Edition

Books on electrocardiography seem to possess one or more of several disadvantages for the beginner: the introductory chapters on electrophysiology are so intricate and longwinded that the reader's interest is early drowned in a troubled sea of vectors, axes and gradients; or only certain aspects of the subject are dealt with, for example, the arrhythmias may be entirely omitted; or illustrations are deficient and frequently situated uncomfortably far from the descriptive text.

For several years I have been attempting to introduce fourth year students to the comparatively easy technique of interpreting electrocardiograms. During this period I have been unable to recommend any single text that deals with the subject quickly and simply and yet is sufficiently comprehensive. This book is an attempt to supply such a manual. Its aims are: 1) to emphasize the simplicities rather than the complexities of the electrocardiogram; 2) to give the reader only those electrophysiologic concepts that make everyday interpretation more intelligible without burdening him with unnecessary detail; 3) to cover all diagnostically important electrocardiographic patterns; and 4) to provide adequate illustrations and in every instance to have the illustration conveniently situated to the reader as he reads the descriptive text. To achieve this last desideratum, the publishers have generously waived publishing conventions and given me a free hand in the arrangement and spacing of illustrations and text.

This book is designed for those approaching electrocardiography from the point of view of the clinician. It is hoped that it will enable the beginner to acquire a rapid but thorough grasp of a sophisticated yet simple discipline.

H. J. L. M.

Acknowledgments

It is a great pleasure to acknowledge my indebtedness:

To Marcie Etheridge Perry and Raymond Rochkind for their excellent line drawings; to Dr. William Schuman for coining the mot juste, electrocardiographogenic; to Dr. Otto Vogel for improving my approach to the electrical axis.

To the following colleagues for providing me with illustrative tracings: Dr. Emory Hollar for figure 165; Dr. Victor Schulze for figure TR-31, Dr. Thomas Ross for figure 151; Dr. Nathan Marcus for figure 245; Dr. L. E. Bilodeau for figure 158; Dr. Joseph Bowen for figure 159; Dr. Leo Schamroth for figure 142; Dr. Roger Sutton for figure 155; Dr. Robert Myerburg for figure 11; Dr. Breffni O'Neill for figures 225 and X; Dr. Alan Lindsay for figure 64; Dr. Carol Kramer for figure TR-14; and Dr. Morris Fulton and the electrocardiograph department of the King Edward VII Memorial Hospital in Bermuda for figures 134 and 224.

To the electrocardiograph departments of the Mercy Hospital in Baltimore, the Tampa General Hospital and St. Anthony's Hospital in St. Petersburg as the sources of most of the remaining tracings; and especially to technicians—past and present—for their interest and zeal in capturing good records of arrhythmias.

To innumerable students and many colleagues throughout the country who have stimulated me with encouragement or criticism.

To the publishers, whose gracious cooperation has now been patient and unfailing through five gestations.

H. J. L. M.

Contents

Introductory Note

Much of electrocardiography is simple, but it does not always provide a clearcut answer. Our knowledge of the electrocardiogram has definite limitations which must be appreciated. In the arrhythmias and blocks it often gives a clear and irrefutable answer, but with myocardial disease there is much less specificity. Every interpreter, no matter how experienced, encounters tracings he cannot unravel. Not infrequently a tracing is "borderline" or "abnormal but non-specific" and must be classified as such—an unsatisfying situation for both the interpreter and the clinician in charge of the case, yet one which should be frankly and humbly faced.

Profession and laity alike are inclined to lay too much stress on mechanical devices in diagnosis. The electrocardiograph is no exception. A patient with a normal tracing may drop dead of a coronary attack five minutes later, while another, with a grossly abnormal tracing, may live on without cardiac symptoms for many years.

The electrocardiogram should always be read in the clearest light of clinical observation. All pertinent data should be in the hands of the interpreter. Ideally the clinician in charge of the case reads his own tracings; failing this he should see to it that his interpreting colleague is furnished with full details, including his own clinical impression, for only so will he and his patient derive maximal benefit from expert interpretation.

As electrocardiographic interpretation and clinical observation are, or should be, inseparable, a certain number of clinical notes of practical diagnostic value are included in this primarily electrocardiographic text.

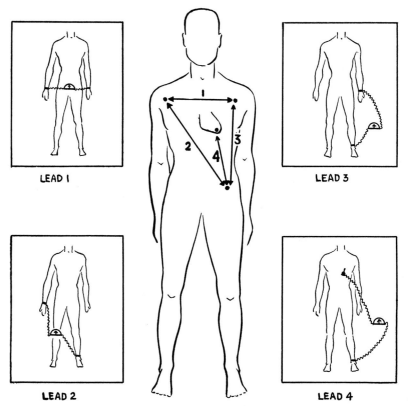

LEAD 1   LEAD 3

LEAD 2   LEAD 4

FIG. 1. The standard limb leads and the original precordial lead

Caution: The double-headed arrows in the diagram are not intended to represent Einthoven's triangle.

1

Electrodes and Leads

STANDARD LIMB LEADS

These are three in number and have been in use for over 60 years. We therefore have far more empirical knowledge of these than of the numerous additional leads more recently introduced. Probably 80 to 90 per cent accuracy in diagnosis can be achieved by inspecting these leads alone. Most arrhythmias and most types of heart block are easily diagnosed from them.

The connections of these leads are illustrated in figure 1. Lead 1 connects the two arms; lead 3 connects the left arm with the left leg; and lead 2, the hypotenuse of the triangle, connects the right arm with the left leg. Each lead records the difference in potential between the two connected limbs. Although the electrodes are attached at wrists and ankle this is purely a matter of convenience—it is easiest to attach bracelets to these parts of the limbs. It is more accurate to think of the potential as derived from the roots of the respective limbs, i.e., from the two shoulders and the left groin. The heart is approximately in the center of the triangle so formed (fig. 1).

It is worth noting **Einthoven's law**, which states, in effect, that a complex in lead 2 is equal to the sum of the corresponding complexes in leads 1 and 3 (2 = 1 + 3). This is a helpful rule to remember when the technician has wrongly labelled the leads. For example, if the P wave is seen to be upright in all three leads, you know at a glance that the lead with the tallest P is lead 2.

PRECORDIAL LEADS

The standard limb leads have two disadvantages: 1) each is derived from *two* points *distant* from the heart and 2) the three electrodes are all in the same plane, i.e., the frontal plane of the body. It is not surprising that we can gain additional information by placing electrodes closer to the heart and moving them round the bend of the thorax to obtain "views" of the heart from different angles. The first precordial or chest lead, introduced in 1932, connected the left leg with the apex beat and was called lead 4 (fig. 1). This was a successful innovation and soon a series of precordial points was introduced whose positions are illustrated in figure 2. Point 1 is just to the right of the sternum in the fourth interspace; point 2, just to the left of the sternum in the fourth interspace. Point 4 lies in the midclavicular line in the fifth interspace. Point 3 is halfway between 2 and 4. Points 5, 6 and 7 are at the same level as 4 in the anterior, middle and posterior axillary lines, respectively.

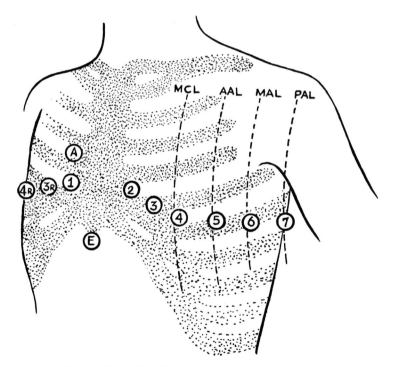

Fig. 2. Precordial points from which chest leads are derived

Most cardiologists employ precordial positions from 1 to 6 routinely. Sometimes it is desirable to take additional leads from further points; some of these are also illustrated in figure 2. Point E is situated over the ensiform process. The atrial lead point (A) is just to the right of the sternum in the third interspace. The locations of further right precordial points, 3_R, 4_R, etc., correspond with the locations of their opposite numbers on the left side of the chest. Occasionally it is desirable to take leads from the posterior thorax; points 8 and 9 are at the angle of the scapula and over the spine, at the same level as 4, 5, 6 and 7. At times, especially for the purpose of unravelling difficult arrhythmias, it is useful to obtain a tracing from behind the left atrium by means of an esophageal electrode; or from the cavity of the right atrium by means of a transvenous wire electrode (6).

In a standard lead the two electrodes are about equally remote from the heart and are therefore about equally important in their contribution to the tracing. When, however, one electrode is placed in one of the precordial positions while the other electrode is on a limb, it is natural that the closer chest electrode should contribute more to the tracing, and the limb electrode less. The limb attachment of such a lead is therefore called the **indifferent electrode** and the chest electrode is referred to as the **exploring electrode**, since it is moved in an exploratory fashion from point to point across the chest. If the indifferent electrode is attached to the left leg the connection is designated CF; if to the right arm CR; if to the left arm CL. According to the precordial point employed a subscribed number is added to the CF, CR or CL label. Thus, for example, lead CF_5 indicates that the exploring electrode is placed at point 5 in the anterior axillary line while the indifferent electrode is attached to the left ankle.

V LEADS

Though the exploring electrode exerts a far greater influence on the tracing than the indifferent electrode, the indifferent electrode nevertheless has considerable influence. It was discovered empirically, however, that if all three limb electrodes were connected, through resistances of 5000 ohms each, to form a common **central terminal**, this afforded a more truly indifferent connection—the potential at such a central terminal was practically zero throughout the cardiac cycle. Thus, theoretically at any rate, such a connection leaves the exploring electrode as sole dictator of the pattern. The hookup of the V leads is diagrammatically shown in figure 3.

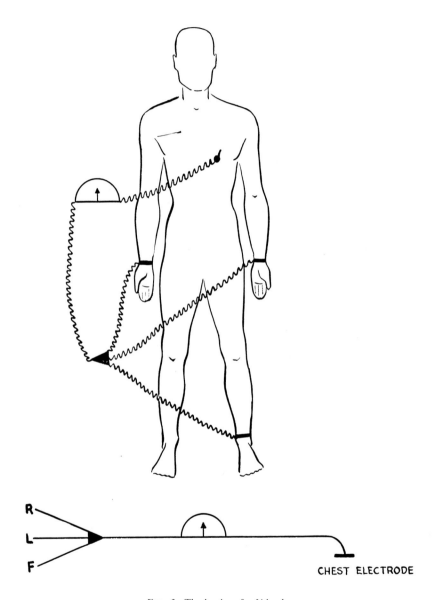

FIG. 3. The hookup for V leads

Although theoretically the V lead connections should give the most reliable precordial pattern, in practice it is not so certain that they always do (2); and at least one authority (3, 4) insists that the CR connection is the most satisfactory. At any rate, it is worth appreciating the expected differences between the various precordial connections. These may best be summarized by stating that the CR leads tend to emphasize positive (upright) deflections, while the CF leads lend emphasis to negative (downward). The pattern of V leads usually lies somewhere in between. It may sometimes be useful to take advantage of the "emphasizing" tendencies of the CR and CF connections, rather than to rely slavishly on the V leads because they are theoretically superior. Such employment of the CR or CF leads may be likened to the use of a magnifying glass to detect otherwise invisible or questionable changes. CL connections found little favor or use until a modified CL ("MCL") hookup came into its own for the constant monitoring of patients in coronary care units (see chapter 8).

Figure 4 illustrates the difference between CF and V tracings taken from identical precordial positions. The difference in respective T waves is readily apparent.

aV LEADS

The standard limb leads are strictly **bipolar**, representing as they do the difference in potential between two points. CF, CR and CL leads

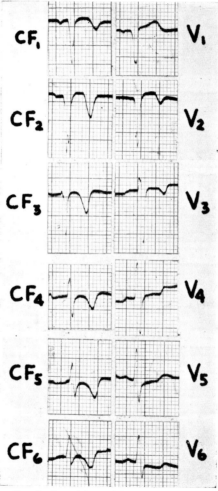

FIG. 4. Compàrison of CF and V tracings on the same patient, taken from identical precordial points.

are also clearly bipolar, in that they too record the difference in potential between two points. In the standard leads the two points involved exert approximately equal influences, whereas in the C leads, as stated above, the precordial point is more influential than the more distant limb connection. With the V leads comes the virtual exclusion of this distant influence because the central terminal shows practically zero potential throughout the heart cycle. They are therefore referred to as **unipolar** precordial leads. From this development it is only a short step to the unipolar *limb* leads. By using the central terminal as the indifferent connection and placing the exploring electrode on one limb, the resulting tracing might well be expected to record the potential at the root of the "explored" limb exclusively. Such leads are labeled VR, VL and VF according to the limb with which the exploring electrode is connected. The connections of VF are diagrammatically shown in figure 5 A. The deflections in such a lead are small; but the amplitude of complexes in such leads can be materially increased by disconnecting the central terminal attachment to the explored limb (fig. 5 B). This device increases the

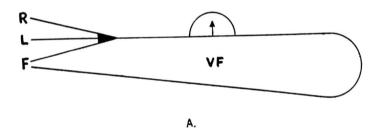

A.

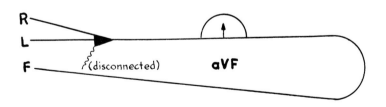

B.

FIG. 5. A. The hookup for lead V̇F. B. The hookup for augmented VF (aVF).

size of the deflections (thus making them more readable) without significantly altering their shape. This *augmentation* of potential is designated by a prefixed "a"—aVR, aVL, aVF.

RELATION OF BIPOLAR TO UNIPOLAR LIMB LEADS

In a sense, the unipolar limb leads are the algebraic bricks of which the bipolar leads are built. Lead 1 represents the difference between aVR and aVL; lead 2 the difference between aVR and aVF; and lead 3 between aVL and aVF.

Now, quite arbitrarily, as originally ordained by Einthoven, the polarity of the electrodes is arranged as in figure 6. F is positive in relation to R in lead 2 and relative to L in lead 3; while in lead 1 L is positive in relation to R. In other words, F is always relatively positive and R is always relatively negative, while L is variable as between leads 1 and 3. The relationships between the bipolar and unipolar limb leads can thus be summarized in the following equations:

$$\text{lead } 1 = aVL - aVR$$
$$\text{lead } 2 = aVF - aVR$$
$$\text{lead } 3 = aVF - aVL$$

The information available from the six limb leads can be deduced from any two of them. In theory, therefore, it is only necessary to take two of the limb leads, but in practice it is valuable to acquire a working knowledge of all six. If only two leads are taken, it has been found that the most suitable and informative pair are 1 and aVF (5).

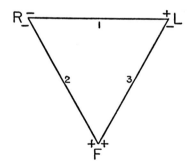

FIG. 6. Polarity of electrodes in the standard leads

CONCLUSION

In a routine screening electrocardiogram 12 leads should be employed: the three standard limb leads, the three aV leads and six V leads from 1 to 6 inclusive. For certain purposes, however, this number of leads is inadequate, while for other purposes 12 leads are quite unnecessary. In following the progress of an arrhythmia a single lead 2 or V_1 is usually ample, whereas in a doubtful case of myocardial infarction it may be expedient to explore additional higher and more lateral areas of the precordium. There should be no rigid routine. While the usual 12 leads are generally adequate and necessary, the number should be freely modified or supplemented by an intelligent understanding of the particular requirements.

REFERENCES

1. Douglas, A. H., and Cohen, N.: The vector and algebraic relationship of the CF and V chest leads. Am. Heart J. 1954: **48,** 340.
2. Editorial: Are the V leads always superior? Ann. Int. Med. 1952: **36,** 1548.
3. Evans, W.: *Cardiography*, 2nd ed. Butterworth & Co., London, 1954.
4. Evans, W., and Lloyd-Thomas, H. G.: The infrequent normal electrocardiogram in cardiac pain. Am. Heart J. 1961: **62,** 51.
5. Schaffer, A. I., et al.: A new look at electrocardiographic leads. Am. Heart J. 1956: **52,** 704.
6. Vogel, J. H. K., et al.: A simple technique for identifying P waves in complex arrhythmias. Am. Heart J. 1964: **67,** 158.

Practical Points

Enough variables influence the tracing without introducing unnecessary technical ones. Care should therefore be exercised to ensure that technique is uniform from tracing to tracing and day to day, so that allowances do not have to be made for variations in technique. The following points are of importance.

1. Effective *contact* between electrode and skin is essential. Electrode jelly contains electrolytes and an abrasive; the abrasive is intended to break down the waterproof horny layer of the skin so that the electrolytes of jelly and body may form a continuous conductor. The jelly should therefore be rubbed briskly, not delicately smeared, on the skin before the electrode is applied.

   On the other hand, special jelly is seldom necessary, and Lewes obtained equally good records using a variety of contact substances including handcream, mayonnaise, mustard, ketchup, toothpaste, K-Y jelly and even tap water!

2. *Standardization* should be consistent. It should always, if possible, be full and should be adjusted exactly. When 1 mv is thrown into the circuit the baseline should deflect exactly 10 mm. If standardization varies from tracing to tracing, it may be difficult to evaluate slight changes. Moreover, the interpreter is given considerable and unnecessary extra work if he has to take note of inconsistencies in standardization and make allowances for them.

3. *Placement of the precordial electrode* is often too casual. It should be as exact and constant as possible. For this reason only bony landmarks should be used in locating the precordial points (page 2). Especially in leads close to the transitional zone (page 50 and figure 30), small displacements of the electrode may produce considerable changes in the pattern.

4. *Position of patient* while the tracing is being taken is of importance. He should be lying uniformly flat. If for some reason he has to be in any other position, a note to this effect should be made. Lying on either side, or sitting up, usually alters the heart's electrical axis and transitional zone; thus serial tracings, if taken in a variety of positions, are difficult to compare.

Some common artifacts are illustrated in figures 19–21.

REFERENCES

Bradlow, B. A.: *How To Produce a Readable Electrocardiogram.* Charles C Thomas, Springfield, Ill., 1964.

Lewes, D.: Electrode jelly in electrocardiography. Brit. Heart J. 1965: **27,** 105.

Schnitzer, K.: *Electrocardiographic Techniques.* Grune and Stratton, 2nd ed., New York, 1960.

2

Rhythm and Rate

In every electrocardiogram 10 features should be examined systematically:

1. Rhythm

2. Rate

3. P wave

4. P-R interval

5. QRS interval

6. QRS complex

7. ST segment

8. T wave

9. U wave

10. Q-T duration

A suggested form for recording routine interpretations is given on page 13.

RHYTHM

A glance is enough to determine whether the rhythm is regular or irregular. If it is regular the interpreter should state whether it is sinoatrial (S-A)—as it usually is—A-V nodal (junctional), or idioventricular. If it is irregular a preliminary survey should be made to determine whether there is a definite pattern to the irregularity, e.g., beats grouped in pairs, every fourth beat dropped, etc., or whether the irregularity is erratic, as in atrial fibrillation.

MEASURING INTERVALS

The tracing is inscribed against a background of millimeter squares and every fifth line is thicker than the intervening four. The horizontal span between two consecutive thick lines is $\frac{1}{5}$ sec. (0.2 sec.); the time elapsing between two consecutive thin lines is $\frac{1}{25}$ sec. (0.04 sec.). The basic interval for timing electrocardiographic events is thus 0.04 sec. In practice, if an interval is to be measured, one counts the number of small squares horizontally contained within the interval and multiplies this number by 0.04. It is an easy matter to multiply by 4 and adjust the decimal point. In figure 7 about two squares are horizontally contained between the beginning and the end of the QRS complex; the QRS interval is therefore $2 \times 0.04 = 0.08$ sec. The P-R interval (from beginning of the P to the beginning of the QRS) measures $3\frac{1}{2}$ small squares and is therefore 0.14 sec.

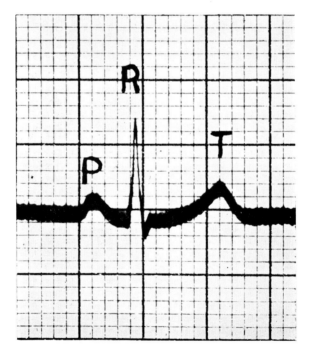

Fig. 7. Measurement of P-R and QRS intervals

SUGGESTED FORM FOR ROUTINE RECORDS

RHYTHM: RATE:

P-R INTERVAL: QRS INTERVAL: Q-T DURATION:

P WAVE: axis:

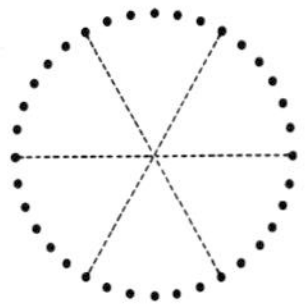

QRS COMPLEX:
    axis:
    Q waves:
    —

ST SEGMENT:

T WAVE: axis:

U WAVE:

IMPRESSIONS:
    (1)
    (2)
    (3)
    (4)

COMMENT:

ESTIMATING RATE

Most electrocardiographic paper conveniently provides marginal markers at 3-sec. intervals. On such records the simplest and quickest method for estimating rate is to count the number of cardiac cycles in 6 sec. and multiply by 10.

When such markers are not available, we use the thick lines as points of reference. As there are 300 fifths of a second in a minute (5×60), it is only necessary to determine the number of fifths of a second between consecutive beats (if the rhythm is regular) and divide this number into 300. For convenience we select a complex which coincides with a thick line and then count the number of fifths elapsing before the same complex recurs. The QRS complex is usually employed, but it is obvious that any wave will serve provided the rhythm is normal and regular. Should there be only $\frac{1}{5}$ sec. between consecutive beats the rate would be 300; if $\frac{2}{5}$, 150; if $\frac{3}{5}$, 100; and so on. Table 1 gives the rates prevailing if from 1 to 10 fifths elapse between consecutive beats. For rates between 30 and 100 it is obvious that reasonably accurate approximations can be made at a glance.

In the second example (b) in figure 8, the QRS marked x coincides with a thick line. There are then $6\frac{1}{2}$ fifths of a second (thick lines) before the next QRS is reached. Thus the rate will obviously lie about halfway between 50 and 43 and may be called 46 or 47 with conviction that the approximation is within 1 or 2 beats of the actual rate. This method is obviously quite accurate enough for all practical purposes, and the slower the rate the more accurate the approximation. For even greater accuracy the intermediate figures provided in the guide in figure 9 may be employed. (These figures are obtained by dividing into 1500 the number of 25ths of a second elapsing between consecutive beats.)

When the rate is over 100 the margin of error rapidly increases and, to determine the rate more accurately, it is better to count the number of cardiac cycles occurring in 5, 6 or 10 sec. and multiply the number by 12, 10 or 6. This method must also be adopted, regardless of the rate, when the rhythm is irregular. Figure 10 illustrates this method for estimating a rapid rate.

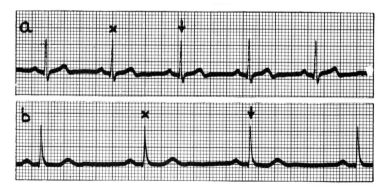

FIG. 8. Estimation of heart rate (two examples). See text and figure 9

TABLE 1

With This Number of Fifths between Consecutive QRS Complexes	The Rate Is:
1	300
2	150
3	100
4	75
5	60
6	50
7	43
8	37
9	33
10	30

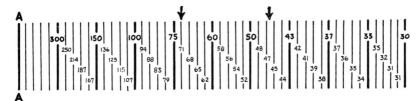

FIG. 9. Guide for rapid estimation of heart rate. In any tracing select a QRS complex that coincides with a thick line (e.g., those marked x in the two examples in fig. 8). This thick line is represented by the first thick line, AA, in the guide above. Note with which line the next QRS in the tracing coincides (arrows in fig. 8) and read off the rate from the corresponding line of the guide: first arrow, rate 71 (tracing a); second arrow, rate 46 (tracing b). NOTE: UNLIKE MANY MANUFACTURERS' RULERS, THIS GUIDE IS NOT DRAWN ON THE SAME SCALE AS THE CLINICAL TRACING AND IS OBVIOUSLY *NOT* INTENDED FOR DIRECT APPLICATION TO IT. IT IS A DIAGRAM *REPRESENTING* THE LINES IN THE TRACING AND IS INTENDED AS AN AID TO MEMORIZING KEY FIGURES.

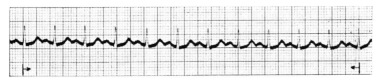

FIG. 10. Estimation of rapid rates. In the 5 sec. between the two markers, there are 11 cardiac cycles. The rate is therefore $11 \times 12 = 132$ per minute.

3

Complexes and Intervals

When a complex is partly above the baseline and partly below it, it is **diphasic** or **biphasic.** When its excursions above and below the line are approximately equal, it is **isodiphasic** or **equiphasic.**

P WAVE

This is the first wave of the electrocardiogram and represents the spread of the electrical impulse through the atria (**activation** or **depolarization** of atria). It is normally upright in leads 1 and 2 but is frequently diphasic or inverted in lead 3. It is normally inverted in aVR and upright in aVF. It is variable in the other leads. Its amplitude should not exceed 2 or 3 mm. in any lead, and its normal contour is gently rounded—not pointed or notched.

Abnormalities that should be looked for are, therefore:

1. *Inversion* in leads where the P wave is normally upright, or the presence of an upright P wave in aVR (where it should be inverted); such changes are usually found in conditions where the impulse travels through the atria by an unorthodox path—as in ectopic atrial or A-V nodal rhythms (fig. 11 C).

2. *Increased amplitude:* this usually indicates atrial hypertrophy or dilation and is found especially in A-V valve disease, hypertension, cor pulmonale, and congenital heart disease.

3. *Increased width:* this usually indicates left atrial enlargement or diseased atrial muscle. The normal P wave does not exceed 0.11 sec. in duration.

4. *Diphasicity:* an important sign of left atrial enlargement when the second half of the P wave is significantly negative in lead 3 or V_1 (see fig. 233 B, page 285).

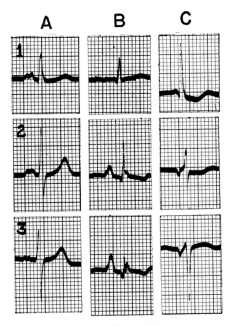

FIG. 11. Abnormal **P waves**. A. **P-mitrale**;
note broad, notched P waves taller in lead 1
than in lead 3. B. **P-pulmonale**; note flat P in
lead 1 with tall, pointed P wave in leads 2 and 3.
C. **A-V nodal rhythm**; note inverted P in leads
2 and 3 with short P-R interval.

5. *Notching:* when the left atrium is mainly involved (as in mitral
   disease) the P wave often becomes wide and notched and is taller
   in lead 1 than in lead 3—**P-mitrale** (fig. 11 A). Notching is considered significant when the distance between peaks exceeds
   0.04 sec.
6. *Peaking:* right atrial strain usually produces tall pointed P waves
   taller in lead 3 than in lead 1—**P-pulmonale** (fig. 11 B).
7. *Absence* of P waves: this occurs in some A-V nodal rhythms and in
   S-A block.

In summary, P waves are:

> Normally upright in 1, 2 and aVF
> Normally inverted in aVR
> Variable in 3, aVL and chest leads

Tₚ WAVE

This wave, formerly called Ta (30), represents repolarization of the atria, and is in the direction opposite to the P wave—if the P wave is upright it is inverted, and vice versa (fig. 12 C). It is usually invisible because it coincides with the QRS complex. It can best be seen in complete A-V block, where the P waves are not followed by QRS complexes and there is consequently an opportunity for the T_p wave to show itself.

P-R INTERVAL

This is measured from the *beginning* of the P wave to the *beginning* of the QRS complex. It measures the time taken by the impulse to travel all the way from the S-A node to the ventricular muscle fibers, and this is normally from 0.12 to 0.20 sec. It is customary to examine several intervals and record that which appears the longest. Other things being equal, the interval varies with heart rate, being shorter at faster rates. But this does not always hold true. If the conducting system is diseased or affected by digitalis, the P-R may lengthen as the rate increases. Similarly, if the atria are paced artificially the P-R increases as the paced rate quickens (5). The P-R is proportionately shorter in children, averaging 0.11 sec. at 1 year, 0.13 at 6 and 0.14 at 12 years. An interval prolonged beyond normal limits is regarded as evidence of A-V block (fig. 12 C).

At relatively slow rates a few apparently normal people, with no evidence of heart disease, have been found to have intervals ranging considerably above 0.20 sec. (32). In a group of over 67,000 apparently healthy airmen, 0.52 per cent were found to have prolonged P-R intervals (4). Most of these prolongations (80 per cent) ranged from 0.21 to 0.24 sec., while in the remaining minority the P-R interval ranged up to 0.39 sec. In another study, 59 of 19,000 healthy aircrew applicants (0.31 per cent) had P-R intervals of 0.24 sec. or more (7). Standing often reduces such prolonged P-R intervals to normal.

P-R prolongation is more likely to be a pointer to otherwise latent rheumatic or coronary disease, but one must not brand an individual as a "cardiac" whose only stigma is an unconventionally long P-R interval. Obviously it is a signal for a thorough search to exclude cardiac abnormality, but if none is found, the heart should be acquitted with reservation.

Biological values do not submit to arithmetical laws, and one must bear in mind all the physiological factors that may influence P-R duration. An elephantine man with a correspondingly large heart will have

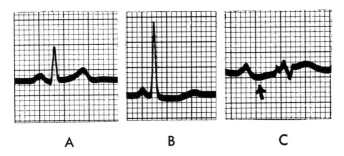

Fig. 12. **P-R intervals.** A. Normal interval of 0.14 sec. B. Short P-R interval of 0.10 sec., from a hypertensive patient shortly after an episode of atrial flutter. C. Prolonged P-R interval of 0.30 sec.; note shallowly inverted T_p wave (arrow) immediately following P wave.

a longer interval than a petite woman less than half his size. She may have true block with an interval of only 0.19, while he may well have a normal duration of 0.21 sec. Biological variations too often are lost sight of in attempting to regiment natural values.

The P-R interval is abnormally short when the impulse originates in the A-V node (fig. 11 C) instead of the S-A node, and also when the passage of the impulse to the ventricle is accelerated as in the Wolff-Parkinson-White syndrome. A short P-R interval is also sometimes seen as a normal variation (fig. 12 B); but this combination (normal P, short P-R and normal QRS) is perhaps not so benign as might be thought, because it is found often in association with hypertension (8) and with the tendency to develop paroxysms of tachycardia (6).

In summary, the P-R interval is

Prolonged

(a) In A-V block (p. 199) due to coronary disease, rheumatic disease, etc.
(b) In some cases of hyperthyroidism
(c) As a rare normal variation

Shortened

(a) In A-V nodal and low atrial rhythms (p. 153)
(b) In Wolff-Parkinson-White syndrome (p. 185)
(c) In Lown-Ganong-Levine syndrome (p. 159)
(d) In glycogen storage disease
(e) In some hypertensive patients
(f) As a normal variation

QRS COMPLEX

This complex is the most important in the electrocardiogram, as it represents spread of the impulse through the ventricular muscle (**activation** or **depolarization** of ventricles).

Proper labelling of the component waves of this complex must first be mastered (fig. 13):

1. If the first deflection is downward (negative) it is a **Q wave.**
2. The first upright deflection is an **R wave,** whether or not it is preceded by a Q.
3. A negative deflection following an R wave is an **S wave.**
4. Subsequent excursions above the line are labelled successively R′, R″, etc.; similarly later negative excursions are labelled S′, S″, and so on.

If the QRS complex consists exclusively of an R wave, the points at which the complex begins and ends are labelled Q and S, respectively, though there are no actual Q or S *waves.* When the complex consists exclusively of a Q wave it is described as a QS complex. A word-saving convention is the use of small and large letters to signify the relative sizes of the component waves. Thus, in figure 13, (c) is conveniently labelled qRs, which is quicker and simpler for the reader's eye than "a small Q, a tall R and a small S wave." In the figure (a) would be

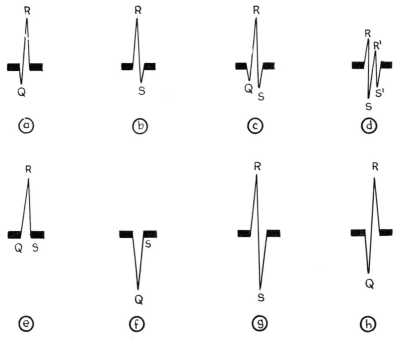

FIG. 13. Labelled QRS complexes (see text)

labelled qR, (b) Rs, (g) RS, (h) QR, and so on. The term "QRS complex" may always be used as a sort of collective noun to describe the ventricular complex no matter what waves actually compose it. Thus all the examples in figure 18 may also quite correctly be labelled QRS.

In interpreting the QRS complexes there are at least six features that should be routinely inspected:

1. Their *duration* (the QRS interval)
2. Their *amplitude* (or "voltage")
3. The presence of Q *waves* (or equivalents)
4. Their *electrical axis* in the frontal plane (limb leads)
5. The relative prominence of the component waves in the precordial leads, V_1 to V_6, noting the *transitional zone*
6. The timing of the *intrinsicoid deflections* in leads V_1 and V_6
7. The general configuration of the complex, including the presence and location of any slurred component

The *duration* of the normal QRS complex is usually given as 0.05 to 0.10 sec., but this is undoubtedly too restricted. At times a short interval of not more than 0.04 is seen in normal hearts, and occasionally an interval of 0.11 must be considered normal. The QRS interval is measured from the beginning of the QRS to its end, and is usually estimated in the standard limb leads. The chest leads frequently display a slightly longer QRS spread (0.01 or 0.02 sec. longer) than the standard leads; the explanation for this is not clear. A measurement of 0.12 sec. or more is indicative of abnormal intraventricular conduction and usually means block of one of the bundle branches or a ventricular arrhythmia.

The *amplitude* of the QRS complexes has wide normal limits. It is generally agreed that, if the total amplitude (above and below the isoelectric line) is 5 mm. or less in all three standard leads, it is too low to be healthy; such low voltage is seen in diffuse coronary disease, cardiac failure, pericardial effusion, myxedema, primary amyloidosis and any other conditions producing widespread myocardial damage. It is also found in emphysema, generalized edema and obesity. The minimal normal QRS amplitude in precordial leads waxes and wanes from right to left across the chest, being generally accepted as 5 mm. in V_1 and V_6, 7 mm. in V_2 and V_5 and 9 mm. in V_3 and V_4.

It is more difficult to set an arbitrary upper limit to normal voltage. Amplitudes up to 20 or even 30 mm. are occasionally seen in lead 2 in normal hearts, while the generally accepted maximum in a precordial lead is 25 to 30 mm.

The amplitude or "voltage" recorded on the tracing is dependent on many factors besides the health of the heart; for example, the distance of the heart from the recording electrode (as determined by size of chest, thickness of chest wall, presence of emphysema, etc.) profoundly affects the size of the recorded deflections. Such factors must receive due consideration before the voltage of any complex is judged too high or too low.

The significance of *Q waves* is one of the most important, and sometimes the most difficult, assessments in the tracing. Size is important, and yet a diminutive Q wave of less than 1 mm. may have real significance, while a QS complex of 10 mm. in certain leads may sometimes be within normal limits. A small narrow Q wave of 1 or 2 mm. is a normal finding in leads 1, aVL and aVF, and in chest leads over the left ventricle, e.g., V_5. Indeed, the absence of the expected small Q waves in these leads may be an abnormal sign (10). On the other hand, deep QS or Qr complexes are a perfectly normal finding in aVR, and QS complexes are occasionally found normally in lead 3 and in leads V_1 and V_2. The Q wave should not be more than 0.03 sec. in width. To gauge their importance Q waves must be viewed in the light of the overall picture and one must take into account 1) their depth, 2) their width, 3) the leads in which they appear and, most important, 4) the clinical setting.

ST SEGMENT

This segment is that part of the tracing immediately succeeding the QRS complex (fig. 14). The point at which it "takes off" from the QRS is called the J (junction) point. Two features of the ST segment should

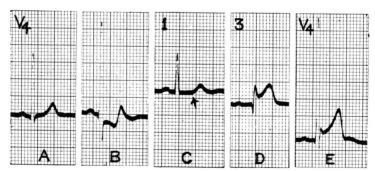

FIG. 14. **ST segments.** A. Normal. B. Same lead, same patient as A; 2 min. after exercise, showing ST depression. C. ST segment is minimally depressed (certainly less than 0.5 mm.) but is horizontal and forms a rather sharp-angled junction with proximal limb of T wave (compare with A). D. ST elevation from myocardial injury (acute infarction). E. ST elevation as a normal variant in a healthy Negro.

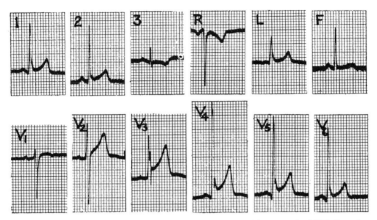

FIG. 15. From a normal Negro man of 29 years. Note marked ST elevation in precordial leads, especially V_3 and V_4.

be observed: 1) its *level* relative to the baseline, i.e., whether it is elevated above or depressed below the T-P segment, and 2) its *shape*.

Normally it is on the same level as the T-P segment, i.e., it is **isoelectric**, or only slightly above or below it. It is sometimes normally elevated not more than 1 mm. in the standard leads, and even 2 mm. in some of the chest leads; it is never normally depressed more than half a millimeter or so. An interesting exception is sometimes observed, particularly in healthy young Negroes (12, 13) where the ST segments may be markedly elevated (sometimes as much as 4 mm.) in one or more precordial leads (fig. 15).

In shape the ST segment normally curves gently and imperceptibly into the proximal limb of the T wave. It should not form a sharp angle with this limb, nor should it pursue a frankly horizontal course. Horizontality of the ST segment, which is highly suspicious of myocardial ischemia, has been called "plane depression" (fig. 14 C).

T WAVE

The T wave represents the recovery period of the ventricles, when they recruit their spent electrical forces (**repolarization**). We particularly notice three of its features: 1) its *direction*, 2) its *shape* and 3) its *height*.

The T wave is normally upright in leads 1 and 2, and in chest leads over the left ventricle (except in infants and very young children); it is normally inverted in aVR; in all other leads it is variable. Certain general rules govern this variability. 1) The T wave is normally upright in aVL and in aVF if the QRS is more than 5 mm. tall, but may be inverted in the company of smaller R waves. 2) In the precordial leads the tendency to inversion of T waves over the left ventricle (V_5 and V_6) rapidly diminishes with increasing age; and in adult life it is generally considered abnormal if the T waves are inverted as far to the left as V_3. The T in V_1 may be inverted normally at any age (indeed it is more often inverted than upright); and in V_2 it is also sometimes normally negative. In normal hearts, when the T wave in V_1 is upright, it is almost never as tall as the T wave in V_6 (15).

We may summarize the direction of the normal adult T wave as follows. It is:

> Normally upright in 1, 2 and V_3 to V_6
> Normally inverted in aVR
> Variable in 3, aVL, aVF, V_1 and V_2

The *shape* of the T waves is normally slightly rounded and slightly asymmetrical. When T waves are sharply pointed or grossly notched (14), they should be regarded with suspicion, though either of these characteristics may sometimes occur in precordial leads as a normal variant. Notching of the T waves is particularly common in normal children (fig. 16); on the other hand, it is sometimes found in pericarditis. A sharply pointed symmetrical T wave (upright or inverted) is suspicious of myocardial infarction (fig. 17).

The *height* of the T waves is also important. They are normally not above 5 mm. in any standard lead, and not above 10 mm. in any pre-

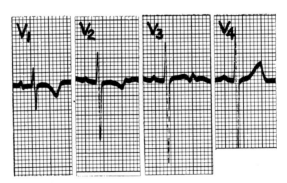

Fig. 16. **T waves** in a normal child. Note marked notching in V_3; this is a common normal transitional form of T wave between the normally inverted T in V_2 and the normally upright T in V_4.

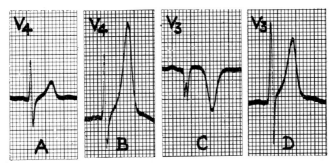

Fig. 17. **T waves.** A. Normal T wave. B. Tall T wave of myocardial ischemia in a patient with angina but without infarction. C. Deeply inverted symmetrical T wave of anterior infarction. D. Tall upright symmetrical T wave of inferior infarction.

cordial lead. Unusually tall T waves (fig. 17 B and D) suggest myocardial infarction or potassium intoxication. Tall T waves are also seen in myocardial ischemia without infarction (fig. 17 B), in certain forms of ventricular overloading (see page 64), in psychotics and in patients with cerebrovascular accidents.

Q-T DURATION

This interval, measured from the beginning of the QRS to the end of the T wave, gives the total duration of ventricular systole. It varies with heart rate, sex and age, and its normal values are most conveniently determined by consulting a prepared table based on the calculations of Ashman (table 2). A useful rule of thumb is that the Q-T interval should be less than half the preceding R-R interval. This holds good for normal sinus rates. However, as the rate slows below 65 the maximal normal Q-T duration falls further and further below half the preceding R-R interval; and as the rate increases above 90 the normal Q-T duration gradually exceeds half the preceding R-R. These points will provide a near enough guide for most practical purposes. The diagnostic value of the Q-T duration is seriously limited by the technical difficulties of measuring it exactly (23).

The Q-T duration is lengthened in congestive heart failure, myocardial infarction (18) and hypocalcemia, and by quinidine and procaine amide. It is sometimes lengthened in rheumatic fever (16, 17, 22) and in other causes of myocarditis (19, 20). Careful measurement shows that it is not lengthened in hypokalemia unless there is an associated deficit in calcium (24). It is shortened by digitalis, calcium excess and potassium intoxication, and may be lengthened by the phenothiazines (21).

TABLE 2

Normal Q-T Intervals and the Upper Limits of the Normal

Heart Rate per Minute	Men and Children	Women	Upper Limits of the Normal	
			Men and children	Women
	sec.	sec.	sec.	sec.
40.0	0.449	0.461	0.491	0.503
43.0	0.438	0.450	0.479	0.491
46.0	0.426	0.438	0.466	0.478
48.0	0.420	0.432	0.460	0.471
50.0	0.414	0.425	0.453	0.464
52.0	0.407	0.418	0.445	0.456
54.5	0.400	0.411	0.438	0.449
57.0	0.393	0.404	0.430	0.441
60.0	0.386	0.396	0.422	0.432
63.0	0.378	0.388	0.413	0.423
66.5	0.370	0.380	0.404	0.414
70.5	0.361	0.371	0.395	0.405
75.0	0.352	0.362	0.384	0.394
80.0	0.342	0.352	0.374	0.384
86.0	0.332	0.341	0.363	0.372
92.5	0.321	0.330	0.351	0.360
100.0	0.310	0.318	0.338	0.347
109.0	0.297	0.305	0.325	0.333
120.0	0.283	0.291	0.310	0.317
133.0	0.268	0.276	0.294	0.301
150.0	0.252	0.258	0.275	0.282
172.0	0.234	0.240	0.255	0.262

Reproduced with kind permission of the publishers from *Essentials of Electrocardiography* by R. Ashman and E. Hull, The Macmillan Company, New York, 1945.

U WAVE

This is a small wave of low voltage, sometimes seen following the T wave. Its normal polarity is the same as that of the T wave (i.e., when the T wave is upright, it too is upright, and vice versa), and the normal wave is often best discerned in lead V_3. It is rendered more prominent by potassium deficiency (fig. 18), and its polarity is often reversed in myocardial ischemia and left ventricular strain (fig. 18). These are the conditions in which its alterations are of most value in diagnosis, but it is affected by numerous other factors; digitalis, quinidine, epinephrine, hypercalcemia, thyrotoxicosis and exercise all increase its amplitude (25, 28).

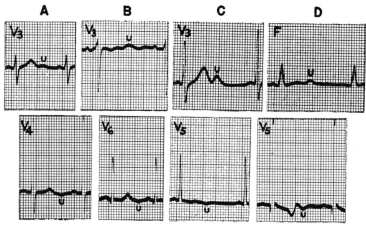

FIG. 18. **U waves.** Upper row—upright U waves: A. Normal. B, C and D. Prominent U waves in hypokalemia. Lower row—inverted U waves: A. Tracing from which this was taken showed no abnormalities except for U wave inversion in several leads; this situation is referred to as "isolated U wave inversion." B. From a patient with hypertension whose tracing showed left ventricular strain including inverted U waves. C. From a patient with coronary insufficiency but without hypertension. D. Note marked inversion of T wave as well as U wave; from a hypertensive.

Its precise significance is uncertain. In the cardiac cycle it coincides with the phase of supernormal excitability during ventricular recovery (27), and in this connection it is interesting to note that most ventricular premature beats occur at about the time of the U wave.

REFERENCES

P WAVE

1. Thomas, P., and Dejong, D.: The P wave in the electrocardiogram in the diagnosis of heart disease. Brit. Heart J. 1954: **16,** 241.

P-R INTERVAL

2. Alimurung, M. M., and Massell, B. F.: The normal P-R interval in infants and children. Circulation 1956: **13,** 257.
3. Blizzard, J. J., and Rupp, J. J.: Prolongation of the P-R interval as a manifestation of thyrotoxicosis. J.A.M.A. 1960: **173,** 1845.
4. Johnson, R. L., et al.: Electrocardiographic findings in 67,375 asymptomatic individuals. Part VII. A-V block. Am. J. Cardiol. 1960: **6,** 153.
5. Lister, J. W., et al.: Atrioventricular conduction in man: effect of rate, exercise, isoproterenol and atropine on the P-R interval. Am. J. Cardiol. 1965: **16,** 516.
6. Lown, B., Ganong, W. B., and Levine, S. A.: The syndrome of short P-R interval, normal QRS complex and paroxysmal rapid heart action. Circulation 1952: **5,** 693.

7. Manning, G. W., and Sears, G. A.: Postural heart block. Am. J. Cardiol. 1962: **9**, 558.
8. Scherf, D.: Short P-R interval and its occurrence in hypertension. Bull. N. Y. Coll. Med. 1941: **4**, 116.
9. Scherf, D., and Dix, J. H.: The effects of posture on A-V conduction. Am. Heart J. 1952: **43**, 494.
10. Burch, G. E., and Pasquale, N.: A study at autopsy of the relation of absence of the Q wave in leads I, aVL, V5 and V6 to septal fibrosis. Am. Heart J. 1960: **60**, 336.
11. Lepeschkin, E., and Surawicz, B.: The measurement of the duration of the QRS interval. Am. Heart J. 1952: **44**, 80.

S-T SEGMENT

12. Edeiken, J.: Elevation of the RS-T segment, apparent or real, in the right precordial leads as a probable normal variant. Am. Heart J. 1954: **48**, 331.
13. Goldman, M. J.: RS-T segment elevation in mid- and left precordial leads as a normal variant. Am. Heart J. 1953: **46**, 817.

T WAVES

14. Dressler, W., Roesler, H., and Lackner, H.: The significance of notched upright T waves. Brit. Heart J. 1951: **13**, 496.

Q-T DURATION

15. Meyer, P., and Herr, R.: L'intéret du syndrome eléctrocardiographique TV1 > TV6 pour le dépistage précoce de troubles de la repolarisation ventriculaire gauche. Arch. Mal. Coeur 1959: **52**, 753.
16. Carmichael, D. B.: The corrected Q-T duration in acute and convalescent rheumatic fever. Am. Heart J. 1955: **50**, 528.
17. Craige, E., et al.: The Q-T interval in rheumatic fever. Circulation 1950: **1**, 1338.
18. Elek, S. R., et al.: The Q-T interval in myocardial infarction and left ventricular hypertrophy. Am. Heart J. 1953: **45**, 80.
19. Fox, T. T., et al.: The Q-T interval in the electrocardiogram of children with tuberculosis. Circulation 1950: **1**, 1184.
20. Gittleman, I. W., Thorner, M. C., and Griffith, G. C.: The Q-T interval of the electrocardiogram in acute myocarditis in adults, with autopsy correlation. Am. Heart J. 1951: **41**, 78.
21. James, T. N.: QT prolongation and sudden death. Mod. Conc. Cardiovasc. Dis. 1969: **38**, 35.
22. Kornel, L., and Braun, K.: The Q-T interval in rheumatic heart disease. Brit. Heart J. 1956: **18**, 8.
23. Lepeschkin, E., and Surawicz, B.: The measurement of the Q-T duration of the electrocardiogram. Circulation 1952: **6**, 378.
24. Lepeschkin, E., and Surawicz, B.: The duration of the Q-U interval and its components in electrocardiograms of normal persons. Am. Heart J. 1953: **46**, 9.

U WAVE

25. Lepeschkin, E.: The U wave of the electrocardiogram. Arch. Int. Med. 1955: **96**, 600.
26. Lepeschkin, E.: The U wave of the electrocardiogram. Mod. Conc. Cardiovasc. Dis. 1969: **38**, 39.

27. Mack, I., Langendorf, R., and Katz, L. N.: The supernormal phase of recovery of con-
    duction in the human heart. Am. Heart J. 1947: **34,** 374.
28. Palmer, J. H.: Isolated U wave negativity. Circulation 1953: **7,** 205.
29. Symposium: The U wave of the electrocardiogram. Circulation 1957: **15,** 68–110.

GENERAL

30. Committee on Electrocardiography, American Heart Association: Recommendations for
    standardization of electrocardiographic and vectorcardiographic leads. Circulation.
    1954: **10,** 564.
31. Kossman, C. E.: The normal electrocardiogram. Circulation 1953: **8,** 920.
32. Manning, G. W.: Electrocardiography in the selection of Royal Canadian Air Force air-
    crew. Circulation 1954: **10,** 401.
33. Packard, J. M., Graettinger, J. S., and Graybiel, A.: Analysis of the electrocardiograms
    obtained from 100 young healthy aviators. Ten year follow up. Circulation 1954: **10,**
    384.

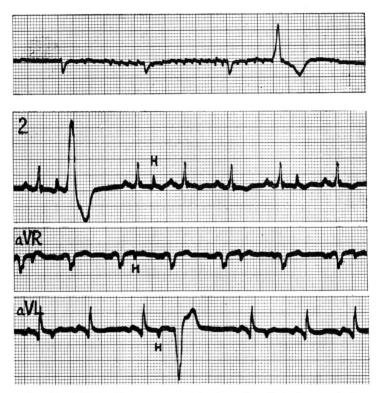

Fig. 19. **Artifacts.** The uppermost strip shows the effect of an involuntary muscular tremor affecting the left arm. The lower three strips are from a patient with hiccups; each lead shows the effect of three or four hiccups, one of which is indicated (H) in each lead.

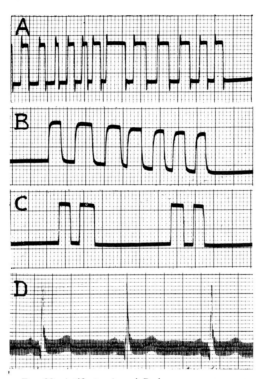

FIG. 20. **Artifacts.** A and B show common errors in adjustment of the stylus—overshoot (A) and over-damping (B)—which can significantly distort the QRS complexes. Proper standardization is shown in C. D illustrates 60-cycle AC interference.

FIG. 21. **Electrodal confusion.**
a. Electrodes properly placed. Leads are as labelled.
b. Arm electrodes (lead 1) reversed:

"1" is mirror image of 1
"2" is 3; "3" is 2
"R" is L; "L" is R

c. Right arm and left leg (lead 2) electrodes reversed:

"2" is mirror image of 2
"1" is mirror image of 3
"3" is mirror image of 1
"R" is F; "F" is R

d. Left arm and left leg (lead 3) electrodes reversed:

"3" is mirror image of 3
"1" is 2; "2" is 1
"L" is F; "F" is L

e. All electrodes rotated counterclockwise:

"1" is mirror image of 2
"2" is mirror image of 3
"3" is 1
"R" is F; "L" is R; "F" is L

f. All electrodes rotated clockwise:

"1" is 3
"2" is mirror image of 1
"3" is mirror image of 2
"R" is L; "L" is F; "F" is R

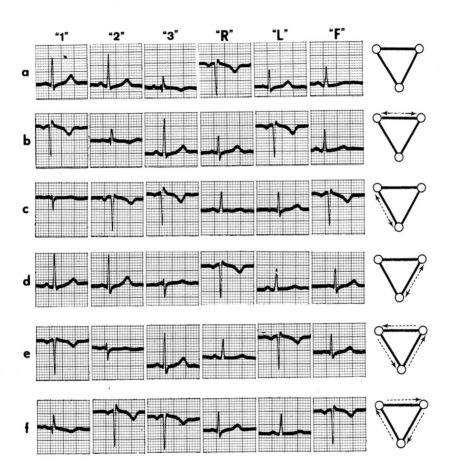

4

Electrical Axis

The orientation of the heart's electrical activity in the frontal plane may be expressed in terms of "axis" or "heart position." The axis may be "normal" or there may be right or left "axis deviation"; and the electrical positions may be "horizontal," "vertical," etc. (see page . . .). But this approach leaves something to be desired. The description, "left axis deviation, horizontal heart," is, like "an elderly old man," both inexact and redundant. Just as we should be precise and say "a 76-year-old man," so we should specify the axis and say, for example, "minus 40°"; this, in a single and relatively accurate figure, combines both "axis" and "position."

The axis can be determined approximately from any two limb leads, but it is most readily and accurately determined if all six limb leads are available for simultaneous inspection. To calculate the numerical axis, one must know the "hexaxial reference system." By taking the three sides of Einthoven's triangle (fig. 22 A), each of which represents one of the standard limb leads, and rearranging them so that they bisect each other, we obtain a "triaxial reference system" (fig. 22 B). If we add to this system three further lines to represent the unipolar limb leads (fig. 22 C), the final figure consists of six bisecting lines, the hexaxial reference system (fig. 22D), each line of which represents one of the six limb leads. By convention, the degrees are arranged as shown in fig. 22 D, with 0° at 3 o'clock and successively greater negative degrees progressing counterclockwise to $-180°$ at 9 o'clock, and with corresponding positive degrees ranging clockwise.

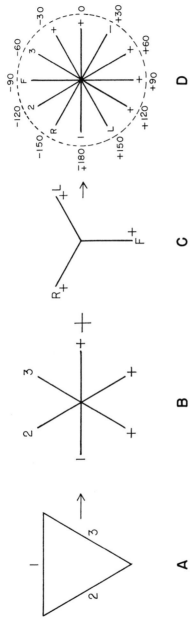

FIG. 22. Constitution of the hexaxial reference system. A. Einthoven's triangle, the sides of which represent the three standard limb leads. B. The triaxial reference system composed of the three sides of Einthoven's triangle rearranged so that they bisect one another. C. Lines of derivation of the three unipolar (aV) limb leads. D. The hexaxial reference system composed of the lines of derivation of the six limb leads (B + C) arranged so that they bisect each other.

One further principle: the electrical impulse writes the largest deflection on the lead whose line of derivation is parallel to its path, and it writes the smallest deflection on the lead perpendicular to it. For example, an impulse travelling parallel to lead 1 will produce the maximal deflection on this lead and a minimal deflection on the lead at right angles to it, i.e., aVF.

To calculate the axis the easiest approach is to look first for the lead with the smallest deflection. In figure 23 A the QRS deflection in aVL is minute, and we therefore conclude that the axis is approximately perpendicular to aVL and therefore parallel to lead 2. A glance confirms that the deflection on lead 2 is indeed larger than the deflection in any other lead and verifies that the axis is parallel to this lead. As the deflection on lead 2 is positive, the axis must be pointing toward the positive pole of lead 2, i.e., +60°. A similar exercise places the axis of figure 23 B as −30°. These two examples are conveniently simple, the axes being situated along the line of one of the leads. Two somewhat more complex axes are illustrated in figure 23 C and D.

In figure 23 C the smallest QRS deflection is seen in aVR, and the axis is therefore approximately at right angles to this lead and parallel to lead 3. As the deflection in 3 is negative, the axis must be pointing toward the negative pole of 3, i.e., −60°. However, the QRS in aVR is somewhat more positive than negative and the axis is therefore leaning slightly off the perpendicular to aVR toward its positive pole, so that a closer approximation of the mean axis will be −70°. Again, in D, the smallest deflections are in leads 2 and aVR; indeed, the algebraic size of the QRS in aVR (subtracting the area of the Q from the R) is practically the same as the deflection in 2. Now if the axis were exactly at right angles to aVR it would be +120°, whereas if it were exactly at right angles to 2 it would be +150°; but it is not exactly at right angles to either because the QRS deflections in 2 and aVR are slightly positive in both. The axis must therefore be leaning slightly off the perpendicular toward the positive poles of both leads, giving an axis of +135°. In E the smallest deflection is in 3, and it is about equally positive and negative; the axis is therefore at right angles to lead 3 and parallel to aVR. As the QRS in aVR is positive, the axis must be pointing at the positive pole of aVR, i.e., −150°.

With a little practice, it becomes easy to place the mean axis rather precisely in a few seconds.

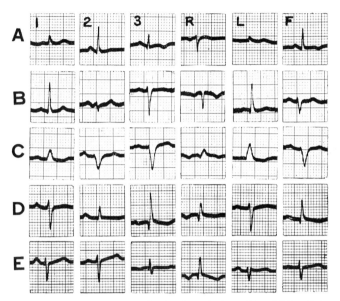

FIG. 23. Illustrating axes in the frontal plane. The QRS axis in each tracing is as follows: A. +60°. B. −30°. C. −70°. D. +135°. E. −150°.

In general, axes between 0° and +90° correspond with "normal axis." Axes between 0° and −90° represent "left axis deviation," and between +90° and +180° "right axis deviation." This leaves the quadrant between −90° and −180° without identity: does it represent extreme right or extreme left axis deviation (fig. 24 A)? This quandary is immediately resolved by using the precise numerical axis. A further difficulty arises from the fact that authorities define the bounds of "axis deviations" differently; according to Sodi-Pallares (4) "slight" left axis deviation begins at +30° (fig. 24 C), whereas most authorities more conveniently place 0° as the rightmost limit of left axis deviation. Similarly, "slight" right axis deviation begins at +60° for Sodi-Pallares, but for others it begins at +90° (fig. 24 B). The Criteria Committee of the New York Heart Association (2) applies left axis deviation to the segment lying between −90° and +30° and right axis deviation to the area between +90° and −90° (fig. 24 B). As normal axes range between −30° and +120°, the most realistic boundaries would seem to be those diagrammed in figure 24 A; this applies "normal axis" to the range between 0° and +90°. "Slight left axis deviation" then applies to the still normal 0° to −30° segment, and pathological deviations of the axis to the left (−30° to −90°) are referred to as "marked LAD." Similarly, "slight RAD" is applied to axes still within the normal range of +90° to +120°, while axes of +120° to +180° are called "marked RAD." Axes between 180° and −150° are conveniently labelled "extreme RAD," and "extreme LAD" is applied to axes between −90° and −120°.

The formulas for axis deviation and heart position thus represent redundant and inexact methods of describing the same thing; they each give an approximate idea of the direction in which the axis is pointing— axis deviation is an approximation based on the standard leads, and heart position offers the same thing based on the three unipolar limb leads. If these six leads are brought together in their proper interrelationship in the hexaxial system, a single precise measurement is substituted for two vague approximations.

These same principles and methods can and should be applied to determine the axis of the T waves, and of the P waves. It is well to plot the QRS and T axes routinely and to symbolize them with a long and a short arrow respectively, as in figure 25. These can be conveniently graphed on a simplified axial system, from which unnecessary lines and symbols have been omitted, as is illustrated in figure 25. Rubber stamps of both the labelled hexaxial system and the simplified triaxial form are useful toys.

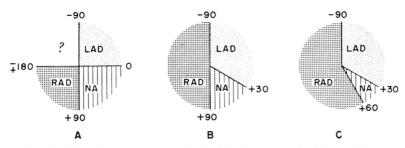

Fig. 24. Illustrating inconsistencies in the definitions of axis deviations. NA = normal axis. LAD = left axis deviation. RAD = right axis deviation. A. Convenient and realistic boundaries of axis deviation (adopted in this book). B. Boundaries recommended by the Criteria Committee of the New York Heart Association. C. Boundaries described by Sodi-Pallares.

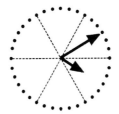

Fig. 25. A simple triaxial reference figure illustrating the plotting of QRS (minute hand) and T (hour hand) on the clockface of the frontal plane. The axes plotted are those of the tracing in figure 23 B.

The T wave axis normally points in the same general direction as the QRS axis; if they diverge by more than 50°, a myocardial abnormality (not necessarily structural) is almost always responsible (1).

One of the advantages of applying the hexaxial reference system is that it teaches us to appreciate the interrelationship of the limb leads and to view the frontal plane record as a whole rather than in fragments. When one grasps this interrelationship it becomes absurd to consider the pattern of a single lead out of its hexaxial context. For example, some writers have stressed the importance of a prominent R wave in aVR in the diagnosis of right ventricular hypertrophy. But, from our knowledge of the mutual interdependence of all the limb leads in the hexaxial reference system, we know that for the QRS in aVR to be mainly positive the mean QRS axis must be *either* further to the right than +120° *or* further to the left than −60°. That is, it may mean either marked right or marked left axis deviation. Obviously it only means right ventricular hypertrophy when it is part of a significant rightward shift in the axis and says no more than that right axis deviation to more than +120° suggests right ventricular hypertrophy.

Axis, as so far discussed, has been represented in one plane only, the plane of the limb leads, the frontal plane. But the cardiac axis obviously has direction in innumerable other planes, being oriented in three-dimensional space. However, the only other plane that our routine leads at all portray is the horizontal plane, the plane in which the chest leads lie. Unlike the limb leads, which symmetrically encircle the clockface of the frontal plane, the chest leads do not encircle the chest but span only a quarter of the chest's circumference. They are sufficient, however, in most cases to determine whether the axis is pointing relatively forward or backward.

CAUSES OF AXIS DEVIATION

The electrical QRS axis may be shifted to the right (beyond +90°) or the left (beyond 0°) in the following circumstances:

Right	*Left*
Normal variation	Normal variation
Mechanical shifts—inspiration, emphysema	Mechanical shifts—expiration, high diaphragm from pregnancy, ascites, abdominal tumors, etc.
Right ventricular hypertrophy	
Right bundle branch block	
Left posterior hemiblock	Left anterior hemiblock
Dextrocardia	(?) Left bundle branch block
Left ventricular ectopic rhythms	Endocardial cushion defects, and several other congenital lesions, both acyanotic and cyanotic
Some right ventricular ectopic rhythms	Wolff-Parkinson-White syndrome
	Emphysema
	Hyperkalemia
	Right ventricular ectopic rhythms

In considering mechanical shifts, note that such disturbances as pneumothorax and pleural effusion usually cause a wholesale shift of the mediastinum, heart and all, toward the opposite side, and do not necessarily affect the heart's axis—they push it to one side without necessarily rotating it.

The reason ectopic ventricular beats and bundle branch blocks swing the electrical axis of the heart as they do is simple. The normal impulse spreads down between the two ventricles and then fans out to both sides, activating the ventricles "in parallel." The resultant direction of spread is therefore approximately in the axis between the ventricles. If, on the other hand, the impulse begins in one ventricle and spreads to the other, thus activating the ventricles "in series," the resultant direction of spread is obviously swung toward the second ventricle. If there is an ectopic focus in the *right* ventricle, giving rise to premature beats, the impulse spreads predominantly from right to left, swinging the axis for that beat to the left. If the *left* bundle branch is blocked, a rather similar state of affairs exists, for again the impulse spreads through the right ventricle first and then involves the left.

AXIS DEVIATION OF P WAVES

With axis deviation of the QRS understood, one can see that the pattern of right atrial hypertrophy already referred to (page 17), with P_1 lower than P_3, is an expression of a tendency toward right axis deviation of the P wave; and similarly the P wave pattern characteristic of mitral stenosis, with P_1 taller than P_3 and P_3 sometimes actually inverted, indicates a shift of the atrial axis toward the left. An axis to the right of $+60°$ is considered good evidence of chronic lung disease.

ELECTRICAL HEART POSITION

For descriptive purposes, the heart's "electrical position," as determined from leads aVL and aVF, is sometimes referred to. The five generally recognized positions are **horizontal, semi-horizontal, intermediate, semi-vertical** and **vertical,** and they are illustrated in figure 26. If the main deflection of the QRS is positive in both leads, the position is called intermediate. If the main deflections are divergent, the heart is horizontal; if convergent, vertical. Semi-horizontal and semi-vertical positions are halfway stations between the intermediate position and the horizontal and vertical extremes.

In other words, horizontal, semi-horizontal, intermediate, semivertical and vertical positions respectively represent axes of about $-30°$, $0°$, $+30°$, $+60°$ and $+90°$. Although the use of these five terms to describe electrical position has little to recommend it, there are times when it is convenient to refer to a heart with an axis in the neighborhood of $0°$ to $-30°$ as a horizontal heart, and to one with an axis between $+60°$ and $+90°$ as a vertical heart.

NORMAL FINDINGS IN aV LEADS

aVR: All three complexes—P, QRS and T—are inverted. This is to be to be expected, since the lead is an inverted stepchild in the hexaxial system—its negative pole is flanked by the positive poles of leads 1 and 2 (see fig. 22 D, page 35). The inverted QRS complex usually presents an rS pattern, but may be QS or QR in form.

aVL: All the complexes in this lead are variable; P, QRS and T all may be upright or inverted, according to the heart's electrical position. If the QRS is as much as 6 mm. tall, the accompanying T wave should not be inverted. Any pattern of the QRS can be normal, even QS when the voltage is low. However, if the R wave is 6 mm. or more, the Q wave should be small by comparison—not more than 1 to 2 mm. deep and not more than 0.03 sec. in duration.

aVF: The complexes in this lead are also variable, depending mainly on the heart's position. The P wave is usually upright but may at times be inverted. Again, as in aVL, if the R wave is 6 mm. or more the T wave should be upright and the Q wave should be relatively small—not more than half the amplitude of the R and not more than 0.03 sec. in duration.

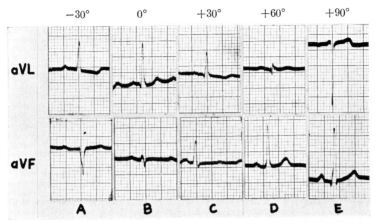

FIG. 26. Electrical heart position. A. Horizontal (axis −30°). B. Semi-horizontal (axis 0°). C. Intermediate (axis +30°). D. Semi-vertical (axis +60°). E. Vertical (axis +90°).

REFERENCES

1. Grant, R. P.: *Clinical Electrocardiography*. The spatial vector approach. McGraw-Hill Book Co., New York, 1957.
2. *Nomenclature and Criteria for Diagnosis of Diseases of the Heart and Blood Vessels.* New York Heart Association, New York, 1953.
3. Pryor, R., and Blount, S. G.: The clinical significance of true left axis deviation. Am. Heart J. 1966: **72,** 391.
4. Sodi-Pallares, D.: *New Bases of Electrocardiography*. C. V. Mosby Co., St. Louis, 1956.

5

Genesis of the Precordial Pattern

THE INTRINSICOID DEFLECTION

Over the normal heart the R wave becomes taller and the S wave smaller as the electrode is moved from right to left across the chest. To understand this it is helpful to consider the patterns that result when an electrode is placed at various points along a single strip of stimulated muscle.

In figure 27 the muscle strip ABC is stimulated at the arrow and the wave of activation spreads from left to right to the other end of the strip. If the electrode is placed successively at points 1, 2 and 3, the illustrated patterns are respectively derived: from point 1 an rS complex; from point 2 an RS; and from point 3 an Rs complex. It is easy to deduce from these patterns that as long as the impulse is travelling toward the electrode, a positive deflection (R wave) is produced, while a negative deflection (S wave) is inscribed when the impulse has passed the electrode and is travelling away from it.

A convenient way to rationalize this finding is to think of the impulse as a moving dipole, i.e., a pair of charges, one positive and one negative, travelling together with the positive charge always leading. This is a crude but convenient approximation of what actually occurs when an impulse travels through stimulated tissue. Let us consider in terms of the dipole what happens when the electrode is placed in the middle of the muscle strip (point 2) and the strip is then stimulated. As the dipole

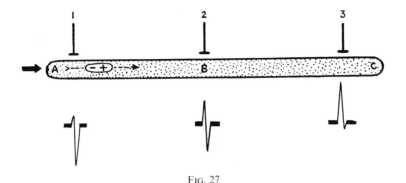

FIG. 27

travels from left to right, the leading positive charge gets nearer and nearer to the recording electrode; as it approaches it exerts a stronger and stronger influence on the electrode and the tracing becomes more and more positive, until it reaches maximal positivity (peak of R wave) at the moment that the positive charge is immediately under the electrode. A split second later the dipole has moved on and the negative charge is now immediately under the electrode exerting its maximal influence. So the tracing makes a quick swing (the downstroke) from maximal positivity to maximal negativity. Then, as the dipole continues on its journey, its negative tail recedes from the electrode and its influence diminishes. The tracing becomes less and less negative until, when the whole muscle strip has been activated, it regains the isoelectric line.

The downstroke which represents the abrupt swing from maximal positivity to maximal negativity is called the **intrinsic deflection**. It is a deflection of great practical importance, for it tells us the moment that the impulse (dipole) has arrived under the electrode. We know that the start of the upstroke marks the moment that the impulse started from the arrow; we now also know that the start of the downstroke marks the moment that the impulse arrived at B. We can thus measure the time it takes for the impulse to travel the distance from the arrow to B. This, of

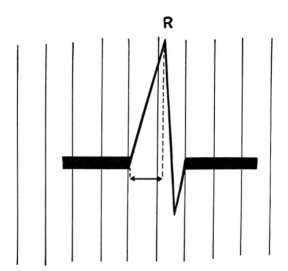

FIG. 28. Timing of the intrinsic deflection. The time
that elapses from the beginning of the QRS complex to the
peak of the R wave is measured horizontally.

course, like all timing, is measured horizontally as illustrated in figure
28. This simple principle has been used for decades in experimental
physiology. Lewis used it to plot the times of impulse arrival at various
points in the atria when he was attempting to prove his theory of circus
movement. Prinzmetal used it even more extensively in his more recent
experiments on the atrial arrhythmias.

In the light of this let us now examine what happens when electrodes
are placed in contact with the myocardium of normally functioning ventricles, either in the experimental animal or in man with the heart surgically exposed. If an electrode is placed in contact with the surface of the
right ventricle, a mainly negative (rS) deflection is inscribed; if placed in
contact with the left ventricle, a mainly positive (qR) complex is registered. For all practical purposes the patterns are the same as those obtained clinically from precordial points to the right and left, say V_1 and
V_5. To appreciate the reason for this one must recall the sequence in
which the ventricular muscle is depolarized (fig. 29).

The impulse apparently descends the left bundle branch rather more
rapidly than the right, with the result that the left septal surface is activated about 0.01 sec. before the right septal surface. The net result is
that the septum is activated mainly from left to right (**1**). Then both ven-

tricular walls are activated simultaneously, but because the right wall is much thinner than the left, the impulse traverses its perpendicular path through the right wall (2) and arrives at the epicardium well before impulses on the left have reached the epicardial surface. Then, finally, the left ventricular muscle is "penetrated," first at the apex and then successively toward the base (3–5).

Now if an electrode is placed over the thin wall of the right ventricle (A in fig. 29), the first impulse (dipole) to influence it will be that traversing the septum from left to right (1); this is travelling toward the electrode and the deflection produced will therefore be positive. The next impulse (2) is also travelling toward A and therefore augments the already positive deflection. From this time on, the only dipoles left in the picture are those activating the left ventricle. These are all travelling away from the electrode A and therefore cause a negative deflection. The wall is thick and the impulses have a relatively long journey, so the S wave is relatively deep. The composite picture produced is thus an rS complex.

When an electrode is placed over the left ventricle (B in fig. 29), again the first influence felt is (1). This is now travelling away from our electrode and therefore causes a small initial negative deflection (Q wave). From now on the electrode is under the influence of the approaching

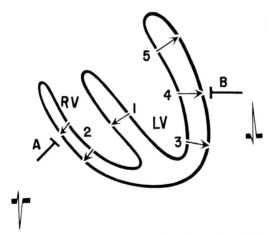

FIG. 29. The approximate order of activation of the ventricular myocardium, and the form of ventricular complex derived over each ventricle.

impulses travelling toward it through the left ventricular wall. Therefore the remainder of the left ventricular tracing is positive, and the composite picture is a qR complex.

Thus over the right ventricle a deep S wave represents activation of the left ventricle, while over the left ventricle itself its activation is represented by a tall R wave. From both sides of the heart the major deflection represents activation of the major (left) ventricle. As in the single muscle strip, the downstroke from the peak of the R wave is the intrinsic deflection and tells us when the impulse has reached the epicardial surface of the ventricle over which the electrode is placed. As the right ventricle has a much thinner wall, the impulse over this ventricle naturally reaches the surface much earlier than it reaches the surface of the left ventricle; i.e., the peak of the small R wave over the right ventricle is reached earlier than the peak of the tall R wave over the left ventricle.

In clinical practice we obviously cannot take **direct** or **epicardial leads,** and the best we can do is to place the electrode on the chest wall at strategic intervals across the precordium. The resulting series of **semi-direct** or **precordial leads** produces patterns very similar to those taken with the electrode in direct epicardial contact. In these clinical leads the downstroke is the analogue of the intrinsic deflection and is therefore called the **intrinsicoid deflection.** This deflection should begin, i.e., the peak of the R wave should be reached, within 0.02 sec. in V_1 and within 0.04 sec. in V_6. If it takes longer than this for the intrinsicoid deflection to start downward, it means that the impulse is late in reaching the epicardial surface of the ventricle under the electrode, and this indicates either that the wall of the ventricle has become thickened (ventricular hypertrophy) or dilated (so that the conducting paths have been lengthened), or that there is a block in the conducting system to the ventricle concerned (bundle branch block).

This application of the dipole concept to the complex process of activation of the entire heart is obviously an over-simplification, though a most convenient and practical one. Regardless of what term—impulse, dipole, electromotive force or vector—is used in describing the phenomena of myocardial activation, the principles enunciated above are helpful in visualizing the train of electrical events.

"CLOCKWISE" AND "COUNTERCLOCKWISE" ROTATION

Between the definite "right ventricular" pattern (rS) of V_1 and the definite "left ventricular" pattern (qR) of V_6, there are transitional patterns—the S wave becomes less deep as the electrode is moved toward the left while the R wave becomes progressively taller. The **transitional zone** is the area in which the QRS is equiphasic (an RS complex), and this usually appears in V_3 or V_4 or between them. In figure 30 five series of precordial leads from V_1 to V_6 are recorded. The first three show normal transitional zones (T): in A lead V_3 shows the equiphasic complex; in B lead V_4 shows it; in C the actual transitional pattern is not shown, but V_3 presents an rS pattern while V_4 shows an Rs; the transition from one to the other has occurred between the two.

The last two series in the figure show abnormal transitions. In D the transition occurs between V_1 and V_2—the Rs pattern is recorded unusually far to the right of the chest. In E the transition occurs between V_5 and V_6—an rS pattern is recorded unusually far to the left of the precordium.

In explaining this we picture the heart to have rotated about its longitudinal axis. In describing rotation about this axis we are asked to look *up* at the heart from *under* the diaphragm. Thus if the front of the heart revolves toward the left we have, from our subphrenic viewpoint, **clockwise rotation.** If the front of the heart rotates toward the right we have **counterclockwise rotation.** Clockwise rotation will obviously move the zone between the two ventricles toward the left so that the transitional zone in the precordial tracing shifts to the left (E in fig. 30), while counterclockwise rotation will shift the transitional zone toward the right (D in fig. 30). Such rotations are not necessarily abnormal.

NOTE ON USE OF TERMS "VENTRICULAR LEAD" AND "VENTRICULAR PATTERN"

A precordial record is not derived exclusively from one underlying area of the myocardium. No matter what lead is used, the resulting tracing is always a composite picture, an electrical resultant of all the many simultaneous impulses, or dipoles, that are travelling in various directions through the whole myocardium. It is true that the area of myocardium

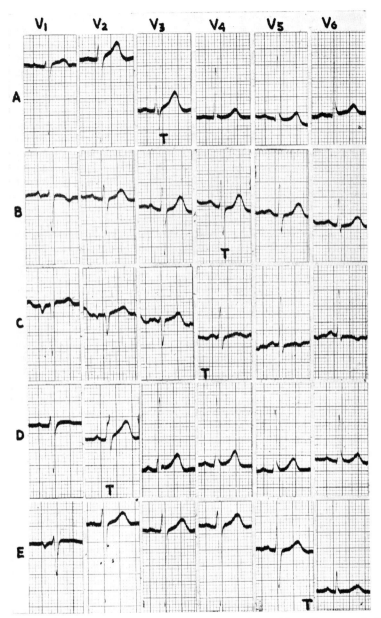

FIG. 30. Transitional zones (T). A, B, C. Normal transitions. D. counterclockwise rotation. E. Clockwise rotation.

subjacent to the electrode may make a major contribution to the record—the so-called "local pickup" effect—because an important factor determining recorded voltage is the nearness of the electrode to the electrical force, and therefore a nearby force will exert more influence than a distant one on the pattern produced. As an example, if the electrode is placed at position 6, the impulses travelling through the wall of the left ventricle are appreciably nearer to it than those traversing the right ventricular wall, and the left ventricle therefore exerts a greater influence than the right; but as long as forces continue to be generated in the right ventricular wall, they will be making some contribution to what we have been calling the "left ventricular pattern." The "vector" electrocardiographers (see below) in particular have de-emphasized the "local pickup" effect and rightly point out that, no matter where the electrode is placed, the resulting pattern is a product of the total electrical forces generated in the myocardium and is not derived from the subjacent area of the heart.

In other words, a right or left ventricular pattern means the type of pattern produced *when the electrode is placed over* the right or left ventricle rather than the pattern produced *exclusively* by the subjacent ventricle. Indeed it is obvious that the so-called right ventricular pattern is mainly derived from left ventricular forces (the deep S wave in V_1 represents *left* ventricular depolarization). Provided one appreciates what is meant by right and left ventricular lead and right and left ventricular pattern, these are useful descriptive terms.

A WORD ABOUT VECTORS

The leads so far described are known as "scalar," and the system employing them is scalar electrocardiography. It seems appropriate to give a word of integration with vector electrocardiography (or vectorcardiography). Students of vector methods have introduced ideas that are helpful and illuminating in our everyday reading of scalar tracings, and the beginner should at least be acquainted with vector terminology and should appreciate the close correlation between scalar and vector methods. The two methods are complementary and should not be thought of as rivals.

Vector is a charged word. It strikes panic into some while it fills others with unnatural pomp and pride. The word is a technical term for force and as applied to electrocardiography obviously means electrical force. As all electrocardiography deals exclusively in electrical forces, all electrocardiography is necessarily vectorial. However, by association and

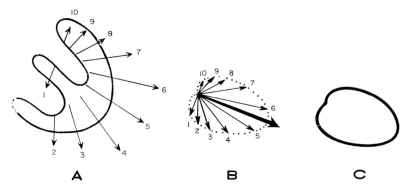

FIG. 31. The **vector loop.** A. Diagram of successive instantaneous axes (or vectors) as the ventricular muscle mass is depolarized. B. Regrouping of the instantaneous vectors in A as though they all originated from a single "center"; the thick arrow represents the *mean* vector, being the resultant of the 10 instantaneous vectors. If the heads of the vector arrows are joined by a continuous line the vector loop is formed (C).

implication, the term has become reserved for that form of electrocardiography in which the heart's forces are represented by arrows and loops, rather than by waves and complexes. *Spatial* vectorcardiography indicates that the arrows or loops are disposed in three-dimensional space—not just two-dimensional symbols on paper like the complexes of the scalar tracing.

Like any other force, a vector has size and direction. Both of these attributes can be conveniently embodied in an arrow whose length is proportional to the size of the force. An instantaneous vector represents the resultant of all the heart's electrical forces at a given moment (any of the thin arrows in fig. 31 A and B). The mean vector is the average or resultant of all the instantaneous vectors (thick arrow in fig. 31 B). The loop (fig. 31 C) substitutes for a set of innumerable arrows a single continuous line and is obtained by joining up the heads of all the arrows; conversely the instantaneous vector for any given moment can be derived from the loop by drawing an arrow from the "center" of the loop to a point at its periphery.

There are two current methods for deriving a vectorcardiogram:

1. The routine 12-lead electrocardiogram can be translated into the necessary vectors from which the loop is artificially constructed. This is the method that Grant popularized (2) and its advantage is that the only equipment it requires is a standard electrocardiograph and a nimble mind. Its disadvantage is that it derives

the vectors only from two planes, the frontal (limb leads) and horizontal (precordial leads), and it obviously can provide no additional information that is not contained in the scalar tracing from which it is derived.

2. The loop may be directly written by means of the cathode ray oscillograph. For this purpose electrodes are placed on the torso in such a way that three leads are obtained whose planes are at right angles to each other (orthogonal leads). Thus each of the three planes—frontal, horizontal and sagittal—is equally represented in the resulting vectorcardiogram. As all three planes are represented, this obviously results in additional information in certain cases, and this is the main advantage of the method. Such a vectorcardiogram may be of particular value in distinguishing between right ventricular hypertrophy and right bundle-branch block, and there is no doubt that at times myocardial infarction can be inferred from the oscillographic loop when it is inapparent in conventional leads. Disadvantages of the method are that the equipment is costly; that the method has no place in that important field of electrocardiographic diagnosis, the arrhythmias; and that, whereas it may be superior to the scalar tracing in the recognition of certain QRS abnormalities, it fails to portray subtle changes in P-, T- and U-wave patterns that are readily discernible in the conventional scalar tracing.

Two further points are noteworthy: the vectorialists themselves cannot agree on the most suitable placement of electrodes for obtaining the most accurate spatial record, with the result that the vector discipline remains at best an unhappily confused one; secondly, it is obvious that the derived loop cannot contain more information than scalar leads recorded with the same electrode positions, and therefore, if one had adequate experience with such leads, one could obtain all the information that the vectorcardiographer can obtain from his loop. Unfortunately scalar leads of this kind have not received the attention and study they deserve.

In summary, vectorcardiography is an interesting and valuable research tool, necessarily of rather limited clinical value; limited because it affords little additional information over conventional scalar leads, because it cannot take the place of conventional tracings in diagnosing arrhythmias, and because of the much more expensive equipment it requires. An interesting survey revealed that established experts in vector interpretation achieved greater diagnostic accuracy from scalar tracings than from the corresponding vectorcardiograms (6).

REFERENCES

1. Grant, R. P.: The relationship between the anatomic position of the heart and the electrocardiogram. A criticism of "unipolar" electrocardiography. Circulation 1953: **7**, 890.
2. Grant, R. P.: *Clinical Electrocardiography. The Spatial Vector Approach.* McGraw-Hill Book Co., New York, 1957.
3. Johnston, F. D.: The clinical value of vectorcardiography. Circulation 1961: **23**, 297.
4. Milnor, W. R., Talbot, S. A., and Newman, E. V.: A study of the relationship between unipolar leads and spatial vectorcardiograms, using the panoramic vectorcardiograph. Circulation 1953: **7**, 545.
5. Scherlis, L.: Spatial vectorcardiography: 3-dimensional study of electrical forces in heart. Modern Med. 1957: p. 172 (Feb. 1).
6. Simonson, E., et al: Diagnostic accuracy of the vectorcardiogram and electrocardiogram. Am. J. Cardiol. 1966: **17**, 828.

6

Chamber Enlargement

With the genesis of the normal precordial tracing fresh in mind, the natural pattern to turn attention to is that of ventricular hypertrophy.

LEFT VENTRICULAR HYPERTROPHY

The pattern of left ventricular hypertrophy (LVH) is what one would predict. If the wall of the left ventricle is thicker than normal the impulse will take longer to traverse it and arrive at the epicardial surface. Therefore the QRS interval will increase toward or to the upper limit of normal, the intrinsicoid deflection may be somewhat delayed over the left ventricle and the voltage of the QRS complexes will increase—producing deeper S waves over the right ventricle and taller R waves over the left (as in the precordial leads in fig. 32). Many criteria have been proposed for the diagnosis of LVH, and they are all unreliable. Probably the best formula so far developed is Estes' scoring system: (1) *3 points* if the largest R or S wave in the limb leads is 20 mm. or more, *or* if the largest S wave in V_1, V_2 or V_3 is 25 mm. or more, *or* if the largest R wave in V_4, V_5 or V_6 is 25 mm. or more; (2) *3 points* if there is any type of ST shift opposite in direction to the QRS, provided no digitalis is being taken (if digitalis is being taken, the shift must be of classical "strain" type—see below—and only 1 point is scored); (3) *2 points* if there is left axis deviation to $-15°$ or more; (4) *1 point* if the QRS duration is 0.09 sec. or more; (5) *1 point* if the intrinsicoid deflection in V_{5-6} begins at 0.04 sec. or later. With a maximum of 10 points, 5 indicates LVH and 4 probable LVH. For good exercise, apply these criteria to figures 32–35, assuming that none of these patients was taking digitalis.

Estes' Scoring System for LVH

1. R or S in limb lead: 20 mm. or more ⎫
   S in V_1, V_2 or V_3:   25 mm. or more ⎬   3
   R in V_4, V_5 or V_6:   25 mm. or more ⎭

2. Any ST shift (without digitalis)   3
   Typical "strain" ST-T (with digitalis)   1

3. LAD: $-15°$ or more   2

4. QRS interval: 0.09 sec. or more   1

5. I.D. in V_{5-6}: 0.04 sec. or more $\underline{1}$
   Total   10

(5 = LVH; 4 = probable LVH)

Unfortunately none of these is entirely reliable. Judging from autopsy correlations, any of them may lead to false-positive or false-negative interpretations. In general, the more of the above criteria that are present in a given tracing, the more likely is the diagnosis to be correct.

"Strain" is sometimes applied when ST-T-U abnormalities develop. Over the left ventricle (V_5, V_6) the ST segments become depressed with an *upward convexity* whose final downward curve blends into an inverted

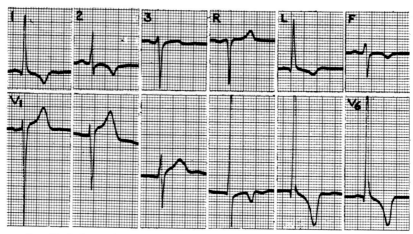

Fig. 32. **Left ventricular hypertrophy and strain.** Note: axis $-10°$ with high voltage of QRS complexes in limb and precordial leads; ST-T changes in 1, 2, aVL, aVF and V_{4-6}.

T wave (fig. 32). The same ST-T changes are usually evident in limb leads having the form (qR) of left ventricular leads. Thus when LVH appears in a heart with left axis deviation, lead 1 and aVL will show ST-T changes (fig. 32), whereas in a vertical heart the ST-T changes will appear in lead 3 and aVF (fig. 34). If the tracing shows tall R waves in all three standard leads, the ST-T changes may be present in all three. A further example of LVH is shown in figure 35. Not uncommonly the earliest sign of left ventricular strain is inversion of U waves in left ventricular leads (fig. 33).

Left axis deviation is not an invariable accompaniment of LVH; indeed, significant left axis deviation implies the presence of myocardial disease in the left ventricle apart from pure hypertrophy (6, 7).

"Strain" is a useful, non-committal term. The exact mechanism that produces its pattern is not completely settled, but there are several factors believed to contribute to it. It is known to develop in those who have shown the pattern of LVH for some time, and the pattern intensifies when dilation and failure set in. Myocardial ischemia and slowing of intraventricular conduction are important among the factors which probably contribute to the pattern.

Along with the left ventricle the left atrium also may suffer. In such cases the P-mitrale pattern (page 17), with a leftward shift of the P wave axis, often confined to the terminal part of the P wave, may be associated with the pattern of ventricular hypertrophy.

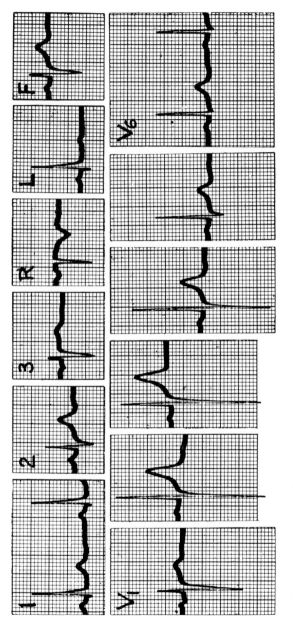

FIG. 33. From a severely hypertensive patient showing earliest signs of **left ventricular strain**—inverted U waves seen in 1, 2 and V4, 6. T wave in aVL abnormally low.

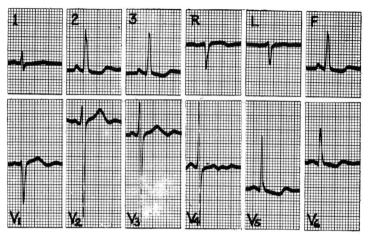

FIG. 34. **Left ventricular hypertrophy and strain.** Note: axis of $+80°$ and therefore ST-T changes in 2, 3, aVF and V_{5-6}. Notice QRS amplitude of over 40 mm. in V_3 and V_4.

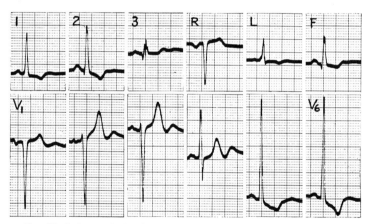

FIG. 35. **Left ventricular hypertrophy.** Note huge amplitude of QRS in V_5 and V_6 with high voltage in all chest leads. Axis is $+40°$, and ST-T pattern is typical.

Much the commonest cause of LVH is hypertension. Less frequently the pattern is found in aortic stenosis, aortic insufficiency, coarctation of the aorta, and occasionally in other conditions.

RIGHT VENTRICULAR HYPERTROPHY

When the left ventricle hypertrophies, the normal dominance of the left ventricle becomes exaggerated and we have seen that the associated electrocardiogram reflects this by exaggerating the normal precordial QRS pattern—tall R waves get taller and deep S waves get deeper. On the other hand, when the right ventricle hypertrophies the normal balance of power is upset and finally reversed, and this is reflected in the electrocardiogram by a reversal of the normal precordial pattern—R waves assume prominence in right precordial leads while deepening S waves develop in left precordial leads.

Most of the criteria for recognizing right ventricular hypertrophy (RVH) center around the QRS pattern in the right chest leads. As the right ventricle hypertrophies, there is an increase in the height of right precordial R waves with concomitant decrease in depth of the S wave and consequent increase in the R:S ratio. If this ratio exceeds 1.0, RVH can usually be diagnosed. There is evidence that V_{4R} is a more useful and reliable lead than V_1, in that it not infrequently reveals an abnormal ratio of more than 1.0 while that in V_1 remains normal (4). In the fully developed picture of RVH, the precordial pattern is completely reversed so that tall R waves (qR or Rs) are written in V_1 with deep S waves (rS) in V_6 (fig. 36). An in-

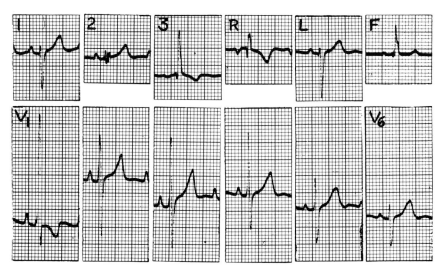

FIG. 36. **Right ventricular hypertrophy.** From a 5-year-old boy with a tetralogy of Fallot. Note: marked right axis deviation ($+145°$), enormously tall R in V_1 and rS in V_6. The P waves indicate right atrial hypertrophy and are typical for P-congenitale.

complete right bundle-branch block pattern (rSr') in right chest leads may signal RVH; and this pattern seems particularly common in the RVH of mitral stenosis (see fig. 233 B, page 285). In the limb leads right axis deviation usually develops and at times prominent Q waves, simulating inferior infarction, appear in leads 2, 3 and aVF (fig. 37). In children, the $S_1S_2S_3$ pattern (i.e., S wave deeper than R in all three standard leads) is a reliable index of RVH (18).

Right ventricular "strain" manifests itself in ST-T changes similar to those seen in left ventricular but in different leads, namely in those over the right ventricle (V_1, V_2) and in leads 2, 3 and aVF. The changes of well-developed RVH are seen in figures 36 and 37. In infants, after the first day or two of life, an upright T wave in V_1 is good evidence of RVH (31).

This full-blown pattern of RVH is much less commonly seen than that of LVH, because the causes of right strain are less common and because it requires a higher degree of strain to produce the mature pattern. In LVH the left ventricle is already the "major" ventricle and as it hypertrophies its majority becomes accentuated, so that early hypertrophy is fairly readily seen as an exaggeration of the normal pattern. In RVH, on the other hand, the right ventricle, starting as the minor ventricle, has a good deal of overtaking to do before it becomes the major ventricle and materially alters the tracing.

A pattern short of the fully developed RVH pattern is more often seen. This consists in rS complexes all across the precordium (clockwise rotation), with right axis deviation in the limb leads. Such a tracing is seen in many cases of emphysema (fig. 38).

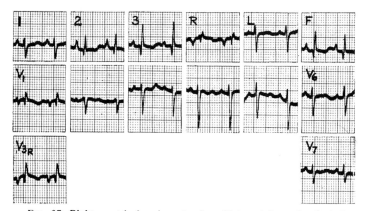

Fig. 37. **Right ventricular hypertrophy.** Note: right axis deviation ($+130°$) with prominent R in V_1; in V_{3R} the R:S ratio is definitely greater than 1.0, while rS complexes are seen over the left ventricle.

In the presence of RVH, the right atrium may also suffer. In such cases the P-pulmonale pattern (fig. 11 B) is added to the pattern of ventricular strain. If pure mitral stenosis is the cause of the RVH, the P-mitrale pattern (fig. 11 A) may appear.

The main causes of RVH are congenital lesions, such as the tetralogy of Fallot, pulmonic stenosis and transposition of the great vessels; acquired valvular lesions, including mitral stenosis and tricuspid insufficiency; and chronic lung diseases, especially emphysema.

Salient Features of Right Ventricular Hypertrophy

1. Reversal of precordial pattern with tall R over right precordium (V₁, V₂) and deep S over left (V₅, V₆)
2. QRS interval within normal limits
3. Late intrinsicoid deflection in V₁₋₂
4. Right axis deviation
5. ST segment depression with *upward convexity* and inverted T waves in right precordial leads (V₁₋₂) and in whichever limb leads show tall R waves

---

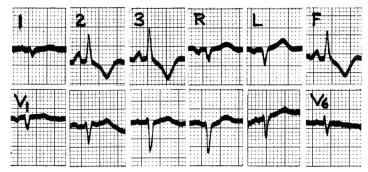

FIG. 38. From a patient with **emphysema.** Note: right axis deviation (+95°) with rS complexes all across the precordium. The ST-T pattern of right ventricular "strain" is fully developed in leads 2, 3 and aVF. The P-wave pattern suggests P-pulmonale with an axis of +80° and pointed, though not very tall, P waves in 2, 3 and aVF.

PATTERNS OF SYSTOLIC AND DIASTOLIC OVERLOADING

The patterns of ventricular "strain" have been subdivided into two types, "systolic overloading" and "diastolic overloading" (2, 3). When the heart has to pump against an obstruction, it is in systole that the strain is felt; when the blood overfills the ventricle, as in aortic insufficiency, the predominant strain is diastolic.

With systolic overloading of the left ventricle, as seen in hypertension and aortic stenosis, the classical pattern of hypertrophy as outlined on pages 56–58 is seen; but when the main load is borne in diastole, as in pure aortic insufficiency, in mitral insufficiency or in patent ductus, a different pattern is sometimes seen; this consists of prominent upright T waves as well as tall R waves over the left ventricle (V_{5-6}) as seen in figure 39.

With systolic overloading of the right ventricle, as seen in pulmonic stenosis or pulmonary hypertension, the classical pattern seen in figure 36 is produced; but when the main load is diastolic, as in atrial septal defect, the pattern of complete or incomplete right bundle-branch block (see next chapter) results. This pattern apparently does not result from blockade of the right bundle branch but rather results from hypertrophy of the basal portions of the right ventricle (30).

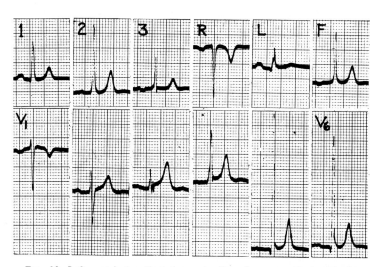

FIG. 39. **Left ventricular diastolic overloading,** from a patient with rheumatic mitral insufficiency. R waves in V_5 and V_6 are unusually tall and are accompanied by tall and pointed T waves. The P waves show P-mitrale pattern, being rather broad and notched with a leftward axis shift to about $-15°$.

ATRIAL ENLARGEMENT

A P-wave axis to the right of $+70°$ (**"P-pulmonale"**) suggests right atrial enlargement (RAE) from chronic lung disease; in congenital heart disease with RAE, the axis is usually not so far to the right (**"P-congenitale"**). Both may show narrow, pointed P waves in limb and right chest leads; but sometimes, when the right auricle enlarges sufficiently to extend toward the left across the front of the heart, the P waves of RAE may be inverted in V_1 and so create the illusion of *left* atrial enlargement (LAE) (see fig. 231 on page 278). In tricuspid disease the P waves may be tall and notched, with first peak taller than second (**"P-tricuspidale"**) (10).

In LAE the P wave is often widened to 0.12 sec. or more, is notched, and its terminal part may be deviated backward and to the left; i.e., it becomes frankly negative in V_1 (1) and may become negative in lead 3 and aVF (**"P-mitrale"**) (11). The product of width (in seconds) $\times$ depth (in millimeters) of the terminal part of PV_1 ("P-terminal force") is used as an index of LAE (19). If the product is more than 0.04 mm.-sec., LAE is indicated. The widened P waves are often notched, the interval between peaks being greater than 0.04 sec. In some patients with pure left heart disease, with no reasons for *right* atrial enlargement and every reason for *left*, a **pseudo-P-pulmonale** pattern may develop (7).

REFERENCES

1. Arevalo, A. C., et al.: A simple electrocardiographic indication of left atrial enlargement. J.A.M.A. 1963: **185,** 359.
2. Cabrera, E., and Monroy, J. R.: Systolic and diastolic loading of the heart. II. Electrocardiographic data. Am. Heart. J. 1952: **43,** 669.
3. Cabrera, E., and Gaxiola, A.: A critical reevaluation of systolic and diastolic overloading patterns. Progr. Cardiovasc. Dis., 1959: **2,** 219.
4. Camerini, F., et al.: Lead V4R in right ventricular hypertrophy. Brit. Heart J. 1956: **18,** 13.
5. Carter, W. A., and Estes, E. H.: Electrocardiographic manifestations of ventricular hypertrophy; a computer study of ECG-anatomic correlations in 319 cases. Am. Heart J. 1964: **68,** 173.
6. Chou, T., et al.: Specificity of the current electrocardiographic criteria in the diagnosis of left ventricular hypertrophy. Am. Heart J. 1960: **60,** 371.
7. Chou, T., and Helm, R. A.: The pseudo P pulmonale. Circulation 1965: **32,** 96.
8. Davies, H., and Evans, W.: The significance of deep S waves in leads II and III. Brit. Heart J. 1960: **22,** 551.
9. Estes, E. H., Electrocardiography and vectorcardiography, Chapter 21 in Hurst and Logue, *The Heart*, 2nd Ed. McGraw-Hill Book Co., New York, 1970.
10. Gamboa, R., et al.: The electrocardiogram in tricuspid atresia and pulmonary atresia with intact ventricular septum. Circulation 1966: **34,** 24.
11. Gooch, A. S., et al.: Leftward shift of the terminal P forces in the electrocardiogram associated with left atrial enlargement. Am. Heart J. 1966: **71,** 727.
12. Grant, R. P.: Left axis deviation. Circulation 1956: **14,** 233.
13. Grant, R. P: Left axis deviation. Mod. Concepts Cardiovasc. Dis. 1958: **27,** 437.

14. Griep, A. H.: Pitfalls in the electrocardiographic diagnosis of left ventricular hypertrophy: a correlative study of 200 autopsied patients. Circulation 1959: **20**, 30.

15. Johnson, J. B., et al: The relation between electrocardiographic evidence of right ventricular hypertrophy and pulmonary artery pressure in patients with chronic pulmonary disease. Circulation 1950: **1**, 536.

16. Mazzoleni, A., et al.: Correlation between component cardiac weights and electrocardiographic patterns in 185 cases. Circulation 1964: **30**, 808.

17. McGregor, M.: The genesis of the electrocardiogram of right ventricular hypertrophy. Brit. Heart J. 1950: **12**, 351.

18. Moller, J. H., et al.: Significance of the $S_1S_2S_3$ electrocardiographic pattern in children. Am. J. Cardiol. 1965: **16**, 524.

19. Morris, J. J., et al.: P-wave analysis in valvular heart disease. Circulation 1964: **29**, 242.

20. Myers, G. B.: The form of the QRS complex in the normal precordial electrocardiogram and in ventricular hypertrophy. Am. Heart. J. 1950: **39**, 637.

21. Parkin, T. W.: Problems in the electrocardiographic diagnosis of ventricular enlargement. Circulation 1962: **26**, 946.

22. Roman, G. T., et al.: Right ventricular hypertrophy. Correlation of electrocardiographic and anatomic findings. Am. J. Cardiol. 1961: **7**, 481.

23. Scott, R. C., et al.: Left ventricular hypertrophy. A study of the accuracy of current electrocardiographic criteria when compared with autopsy findings in one hundred cases. Circulation 1955: **11**, 89.

24. Scott, R. C.: The electrocardiographic diagnosis of left ventricular hypertrophy. Am. Heart J. 1960: **59**, 155.

25. Scott, R. C.: The electrocardiographic diagnosis of right ventricular hypertrophy; correlation with the anatomic findings. Am. Heart J. 1960: **60**, 659.

26. Scott, R. C.: The correlation between the electrocardiographic patterns of ventricular hypertrophy and the anatomic findings. Circulation 1960: **21**, 256.

27. Soloff, L. A., and Lawrence, J. W.: The electrocardiographic findings in left ventricular hypertrophy and dilatation. Circulation 1962: **26**, 553.

28. Walker, I. C., Helm, R. A., and Scott, R. C.: Right ventricular hypertrophy. I. Correlation of isolated right ventricular hypertrophy at autopsy with the electrocardiographic findings. Circulation 1955: **11**, 215.

29. Walker, I. C., Scott, R. C., and Helm, R. A.: Right ventricular hypertrophy. II. Correlation of electrocardiographic right ventricular hypertrophy with the anatomic findings. Circulation 1955: **11**, 223.

30. Walker, W. J., et al.: Electrocardiographic and hemodynamic correlation in atrial septal defect. Am. Heart J. 1956: **52**, 547.

31. Ziegler, R. F.: The importance of positive T waves in the right precordial electrocardiogram during the first year of life. Am. Heart J. 1956: **52**, 533.

7

Bundle-Branch Block

Of the various forms of intraventricular block, bundle-branch block is most common and best recognized. Other forms result from delayed conduction or block in a subdivision of the left bundle branch (hemiblock—see next chapter); from diffuse slowing of the impulse throughout the conduction system of one ventricle; or from conduction disturbances in the ventricular wall. In our current state of knowledge, the terms arborization, parietal and periinfarction blocks appear to have outlived their usefulness.

It is appropriate to consider bundle-branch block (BBB) next for two reasons: first, its patterns are in many ways exaggerations of the corresponding ventricular hypertrophy and strain patterns that we have just dealt with; and second, for those whose main interest is the study of arrhythmias and conduction disturbances (for example, coronary care nurses and anesthesiologists), these are the patterns that probably should be mastered first.

LEFT AND RIGHT BUNDLE-BRANCH BLOCKS

If one of the branches of the bundle of His is blocked by disease, the impulse will travel down the branch to the other ventricle first. Having activated this ventricle, the impulse will spread through the septum to the ventricle on the side of the block and in turn activate it. In other words, the ventricles will be activated one after the other instead of simultaneously, in series instead of in parallel.

There are two main conditions in which the ventricles are activated successively instead of simultaneously: BBB and ectopic ventricular rhythms. There is, therefore, in these conditions a marked fundamental similarity in the bizarre pattern produced: in each there is prolongation of the QRS interval and the ST segment tends to slope off in the direction opposite to

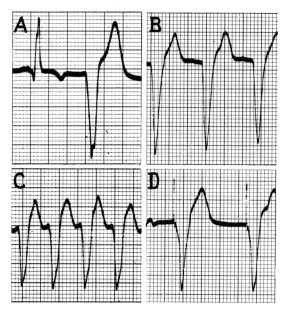

Fig. 40. Comparison of patterns of (A) **ventricular ex-trasystole**, (B) **bundle-branch block**, (C) **ventricular tach-ycardia** and (D) ectopic ventricular rhythm driven by **ar-tificial pacemaker.** Note that each pattern has in common 1) prolonged QRS interval and 2) ST segment sloping off to T wave in direction opposite to main QRS deflection.

the main QRS deflection. A premature ventricular beat, a run of ventric-ular tachycardia and two artificially stimulated ventricular beats are illus-trated side by side with bundle-branch block in figure 40. The similarity of pattern common to all is evident.

In BBB—since the impulse has to push its way slowly through the thick-ness of the septum before the second ventricle can be activated—the QRS interval is prolonged to 0.12 sec. or more, and it tends to be more pro-longed in left than in right branch block. When the left branch is blocked the impulse reaches the right ventricle punctually but it is late in activating the left ventricle. The intrinsicoid deflection over the right ventricle (e.g., in V_1) therefore begins on time, whereas over the left ventricle (e.g., in V_6) this deflection is much delayed (fig. 41A). On the other hand, when it is the right branch that is blocked, just the reverse occurs—the intrinsicoid deflection is on time in left ventricular leads but is late over the right ven-tricle (fig. 41 B). The QRS complex in right chest leads often becomes M-shaped in right bundle-branch block (RBBB) (fig. 42), while wide S waves appear in left leads.

We have seen (page 46) that the septum is normally activated from the left side first. This fact is responsible for a striking difference between the patterns of left and right BBB: when the right bundle branch is blocked, the impulse still travels normally down the left and as usual activates the left side of the septum first. Because of this, the first part of the QRS in right bundle-branch block (RBBB) remains normal and unchanged. On the

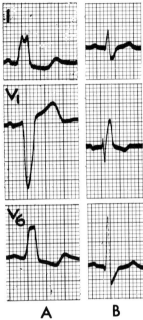

FIG. 41. **Bundle-branch block** (A) left and (B) right. The important leads to study in BBB are 1, V_1 and V_6 (see text).

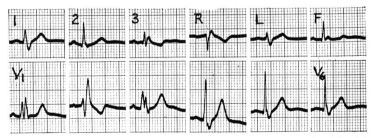

FIG. 42. **Right bundle-branch block**. Note wide S_1, M-shaped QRS with late intrinsicoid deflection in V_1 and early downstrokes with wide S waves in V_{5-6}.

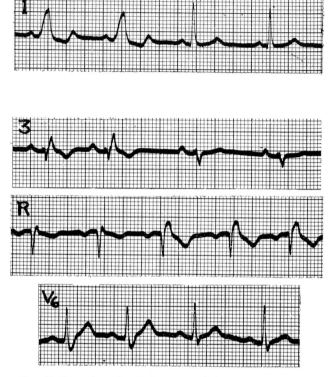

FIG. 43. **Intermittent bundle-branch block.** The first strip is lead 1
from one patient; the remaining three leads are from another patient.
In the first strip the first two beats show *left* bundle-branch block; the
last two are of normal duration and shape. Note that the initial portion of the blocked QRS complexes differs from the initial part of the
normal complexes. In the bottom three strips some complexes show
right bundle-branch block while others show normal conduction; note
that the initial deflection is identical in normal and blocked beats.

other hand, if the left branch is blocked, the normal initial activation of
the septum is disturbed and the first part of the QRS is altered. Normal
septal activation writes a Q wave in left chest leads (page 47) which therefore disappears when LBBB supervenes, and one of the hallmarks of uncomplicated LBBB is this absence of normal Q waves in left precordial
leads.

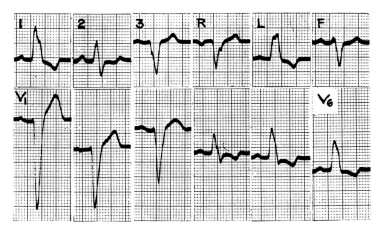

Fig. 44. **Left bundle-branch block.** Note wide QRS (0.16 sec.) with late intrinsicoid deflection in V_{5-6}. There is left axis deviation with the mean QRS axis $-20°$. Note absence of Q waves in lead I and V_{5-6}.

These features are demonstrated in the tracings in figure 43. In the top strip, two complexes showing *left* BBB precede two showing normal intraventricular conduction. Note that the beginning of the blocked QRS is definitely altered compared with the normal QRS. On the other hand, the bottom three strips show intermittent *right* BBB; note in this case that the initial portion of the QRS complex in each lead is identical in both normally conducted and blocked beats.

Characteristic, though less reliable, changes also develop in the limb leads. Leads 1 and aVL usually have the same general features as V6—which is not surprising since these leads have as their positive pole the nearby left shoulder—showing no Q wave and a monophasic R wave in LBBB (figs. 41 and 44), and a qRs contour in RBBB (fig. 41). LBBB is often associated with left axis deviation (fig. 44), but there is some evidence that this implies additional disease besides the blocked bundle

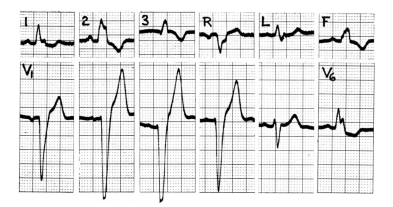

FIG. 45. **Left bundle-branch block.** Note wide QRS interval of 0.15 sec. with late intrinsicoid deflection in V_6. The mean QRS axis is normal, being about +50°. Note absence of Q waves in lead 1 and V_6.

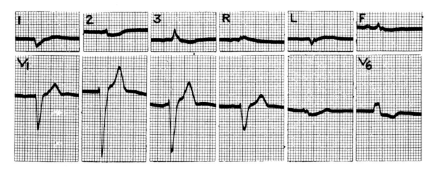

FIG. 46. **Left bundle-branch block.** There is *right* axis deviation, but the precordial pattern is typical of *left* bundle-branch block.

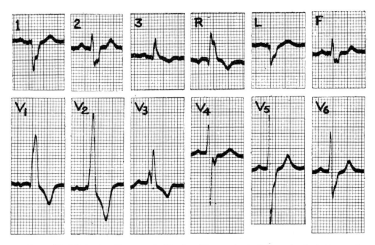

FIG. 47. **Right bundle-branch block** with marked right axis deviation—the "uncommon" type of RBBB.

branch. Certainly it is not uncommon to see a normal axis (fig. 45), and it is even possible to have frank right axis deviation (fig. 46). When LBBB is associated with left axis deviation there is evidence that the prognosis is less favorable than when the axis remains normal (2).

RBBB also can be associated with a normal axis or with right or left axis deviation. If the S wave in lead 1 becomes sufficiently deep, and the QRS complex in lead 3 is upright, frank right axis deviation may be produced (fig. 47). The common type (sometimes still called Wilson block)

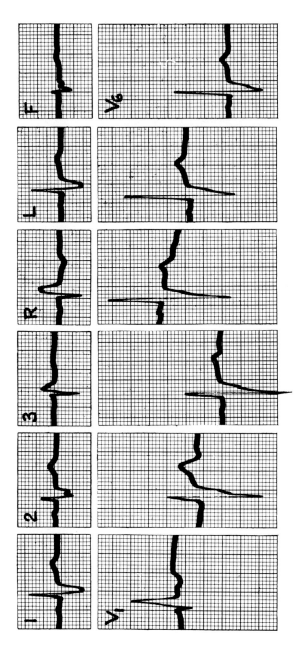

FIG. 48. The Wilson type of **right bundle-branch block**. Note slender tall R preceding wide S wave in lead 1

presents a tall, slender R wave in lead 1 which exceeds in amplitude the S wave (fig. 48). When frank right axis deviation accompanies the RBBB (the "uncommon" type), or when frank left axis appears (figs. 49 and 50), the cause is usually to be found in an associated block of one of the divisions of the left bundle branch (see next chapter).

An interesting hybrid pattern has been described in which the limb leads suggest *left* BBB while the chest leads indicate *right* BBB (fig. 50). Such

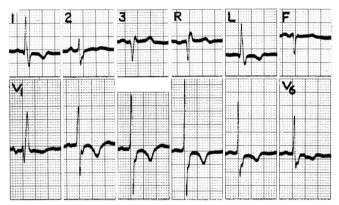

FIG. 49. **Right bundle-branch block.** An example with *left* axis deviation. Note the wide S waves in 1 and V_6 and the rsR' pattern with late intrinsicoid deflection in V_1. Since the T waves in 1, aVL, and V_{2-6} are in the same direction as the terminal QRS forces, these are *primary* T-wave changes (see page 76).

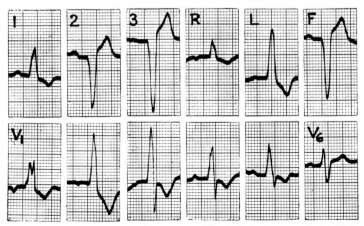

FIG. 50. **Atypical intraventricular block.** The limb leads are typical of *left* BBB, while the precordial leads indicate *right* BBB (M-shaped QRS in V_1 with late intrinsicoid deflection; wide S waves in V_6).

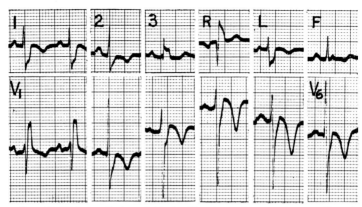

FIG. 51. **Right bundle-branch block** with primary T-wave changes. The axis of the terminal part of the QRS and that of the T wave are similarly directed in the frontal plane and in V_{2-6}.

tracings probably represent RBBB with left anterior hemiblock and are associated with extensive disease of the ventricular myocardium (19).

In BBB the T wave is usually directed opposite to the latter portion of the QRS complex; e.g., in figure 44 the T wave in lead 1 is inverted while the latter part of the QRS is upright, and in figure 48 the T wave in lead 1 is upright while the latter part of the QRS is negative. This opposite polarity is the natural result of the depolarization-repolarization disturbance produced by the block, and the T-wave changes are therefore known as "secondary"—they are part and parcel of the BBB pattern and mean no more than the block itself. If, on the other hand, the direction of the T wave is similar to that of the terminal part of the QRS (e.g., in fig. 51 the T-wave axis in the frontal plane is between −150° and −180°, while the axis of the terminal part of the QRS is about +170°, only about 20 to 30° apart), this is no longer the natural consequence of the conduction disturbance. Such T-wave changes are called "primary" and they imply myocardial disease besides the BBB.

One method of gauging the prognostic severity of T-wave changes in BBB is to measure the angle between the axis of the T wave and that of the terminal part of the QRS complex. Obviously, if the two are oppositely directed (as they are with secondary T-wave changes), the angle between them will be wide and may approach 180°. It is proposed (3) that if this angle is less than 110°, serious organic heart disease is indicated. In figure 48 the angle is about 160°, whereas in figure 51 it is only about 30°.

The pattern of BBB in many ways is like an exaggeration of the pattern of ventricular hypertrophy. Compare A, B and C in figure 52. The differ-

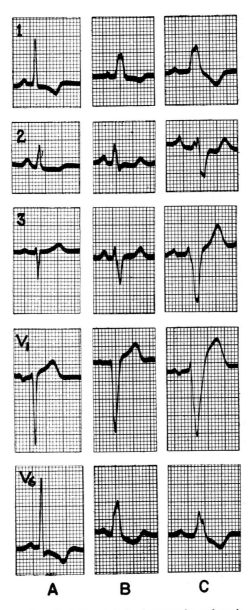

FIG. 52. **Left ventricular hypertrophy and strain
(A), incomplete left bundle-branch block** (B), and
complete left bundle-branch block (C) compared.

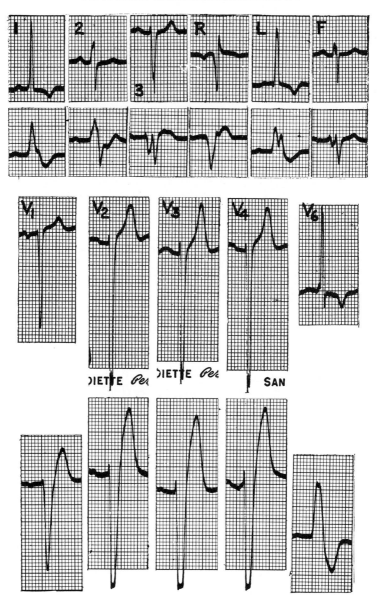

Fig. 53. Two tracings from the same patient, taken two years apart. First tracing (first and third rows) shows **left ventricular hypertrophy and strain;** because of the initial slurring of R wave and absent Q in leads 1 and V_6 some would call this incomplete LBBB. Second tracing (second and fourth rows) shows fully developed **left bundle-branch block.**

ences are that the QRS interval is longer in block, the intrinsicoid deflection over the blocked ventricle is correspondingly later, and the ST-T
changes are more pronounced. The QRS deflections in block are often of
lower voltage and are more likely to show definite notching than in ventricular hypertrophy and strain. One further important detail should be
noted: whereas the normal Q waves over the left ventricle may be present
or exaggerated in ventricular hypertrophy, in LBBB these normal Q waves
are absent. This is because, as the left branch is blocked, the septum is entirely activated from its right side. Figure 53 illustrates how LVH sometimes progresses to LBBB in the same patient.

Sodi-Pallares' criteria (17) for diagnosing incomplete LBBB are initial
slurring of the upstroke of the R wave, with or without small preceding Q
waves, in left ventricular leads; at a more advanced stage, the Q wave is
definitely lost, the slurring is greater and T waves are inverted. All these
features are shown in the first tracing in figure 53.

The designation **incomplete bundle-branch block** has been assigned to
those patterns whose QRS intervals place them in the no man's land of
0.10 to 0.11 sec. with a LBBB pattern (fig. 52 B), of 0.09 to 0.10 sec. with
RBBB pattern (fig. 54).

The problem of secondary R waves (R′) in right precordial leads, in the
presence of normal or borderline QRS duration, is sometimes vexing (24).
Are they due to late but physiological activation of the basal region (outflow tract) of the right ventricle, or do they represent abnormal delay in
right ventricular activation as a result of incomplete right bundle-branch
block or right ventricular hypertrophy? Although there are no foolproof
criteria for separating normal from abnormal, the following pointers are
helpful (18):

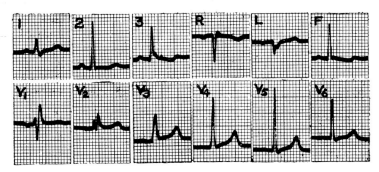

Fig. 54. **Incomplete right bundle-branch block.** Note the salient features of
the right bundle-branch block pattern—wide S in lead 1 with late intrinsicoid
deflection in V₁—but with QRS duration of only 0.10 sec.

1. The R' is probably *normal* if it is present as part of an rSr' complex in V_1 and/or V_2, but absent in V_{3R} or in a low V_1 taken two interspaces below the conventional V_1 position (fig. 55).

2. It is probably *abnormal* if it persists in the lower right precordial leads, or if it is 6 mm. or more tall in V_1 or V_{3R}, or if the R':S ratio is more than 1.0.

LBBB, statistically at any rate, carries with it a less favorable prognosis than RBBB (6, 11, 16). It is obvious, however, that the ultimate outlook depends not on the conduction disturbance per se but on the disease that is causing it. Therefore, in any given instance of coronary disease causing bundle-branch block, the prognosis should be based, not on which bundle the disease process has happened to affect, but one's estimate of the severity of the underlying coronary disturbance. **Intermittent bundle-branch block**, i.e., prolonged QRS complexes present at times but not at others, probably represents a transition stage before permanent block is established.

Left and right bundle-branch blocks occur with about the same frequency (11). Coronary disease is much the commonest cause of persistent BBB. Other causes are rheumatic disease, syphilis, trauma, tumors, cardiomyopathy and congenital lesions. As many as 14 per cent of patients with *severe* aortic stenosis may have LBBB (21). Both right and left block are occasionally seen in apparently normal hearts (1, 5, 8, 20). Among 122,000 asymptomatic airmen there were 231 with RBBB and 17 with LBBB; but in 44,000 under the age of 25, no instance of LBBB was found (4). Transient bundle-branch block may occur in acute heart failure, acute myocardial infarction, acute coronary insufficiency and acute infections, or may rarely result from digitalis or quinidine intoxication.

	Salient features of bundle-branch block:	
Leads	Left Bundle-Branch Block	Right Bundle-Branch Block
V_1	Early intrinsicoid	Late intrinsicoid, M-shaped QRS
V_6	Late intrinsicoid, no Q waves	Early intrinsicoid
1	Monophasic R wave	Wide S wave

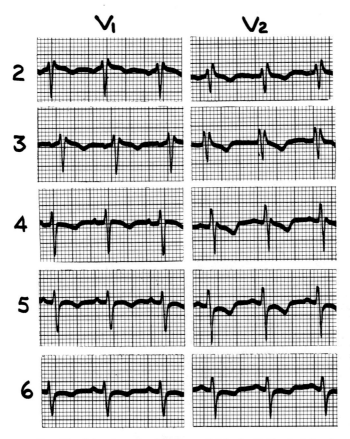

FIG. 55. rSr' patterns in right precordial leads. Notice that the r'
wave, present in the higher interspaces, decreases in amplitude and
disappears in the lower interspaces. (Figures at the left indicate the
interspace in which the electrode was placed.)

RATE-DEPENDENT BBB

At times intermittent BBB is determined by the heart rate. If the rate
accelerates, the R-R interval shortens and the descending impulse may find
one of the bundle branches still in its refractory period so that block of

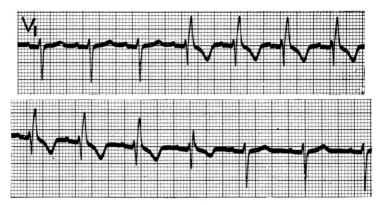

FIG. 56. **Intermittent right BBB**—showing "critical rate." As the rate accelerates in the upper strip from 98 to 102, RBBB develops. In the lower strip the RBBB persists as the rate slows to about 90; the first three beats in this strip show complete RBBB, while the fourth shows incomplete RBBB, and then normal conduction is resumed. As usual, the critical rate is faster during acceleration than during slowing.

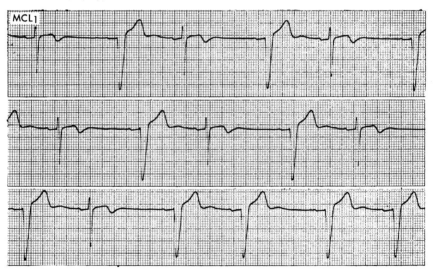

FIG. 57. **Bradycardia-dependent LBBB** (paradoxical critical rate). All beats are conducted sinus beats and they are grouped in pairs suggesting 3:2 sinus Wenckebach periods (see p. 201). Those ending the shorter cycles are conducted normally while those ending the *longer* cycles develop LBBB.

that bundle is registered for a few beats (fig. 56); if the heart then slows, descending impulses may arrive after the refractory period of the branch is over and normal conduction is recorded. The rate at which conduction changes is known as the "critical rate." Knowledge of this phenomenon is of some importance because the appearance or disappearance of BBB is often wrongly regarded as evidence of deterioration or improvement—when it may be merely the result of a few more or a few less beats per minute.

Rarely, the intermittent BBB develops only when the cycle lengthens rather than shortens (fig. 57); it is then referred to as "paradoxical critical rate" or as "bradycardia-dependent" BBB (24, 25).

BILATERAL BUNDLE-BRANCH BLOCK (BBBB)

The patterns of BBBB are varied. If both bundle branches are completely blocked, no impulse can reach the ventricles and the picture is one of complete A-V block. If one branch is completely blocked and the other only partially, the BBB pattern is associated with either a prolonged P-R interval ("first degree A-V block") or dropped beats ("second degree A-V block"). If both bundles are incompletely but equally blocked, only P-R lengthening results with a normal QRS complex. The evidence for BBBB therefore may take five forms:

1. First degree A-V block
2. First degree A-V block + BBB
3. Second degree A-V block + BBB
4. Complete A-V block
5. Sometimes RBBB, sometimes LBBB

Of all of these, only the last is absolute evidence that both bundle branches are involved, since any of the first four manifestations can be produced by blocks other than BBBB.

RSR' VARIANTS AND DOMINANT R WAVES IN V$_{1-2}$

This is a good place to summarize the causes of RSR' patterns and dominant R waves in right precordial leads (24):

Causes of RSR' variants in V$_{1-2}$

1. Occurs in 5 per cent of normal young people (23)
2. Frequently associated with pectus or straight back deformities (22)
3. Incomplete RBBB (fig. 54)
4. RV hypertrophy (fig. 233 B)
5. Acute cor pulmonale (fig. 236)
6. RV diastolic overloading (fig. 227)
7. Wolff-Parkinson-White syndrome
8. Duchenne dystrophy (25)

Causes of dominant R waves in V_{1-2}
1. Occasionally a normal variant
2. RV hypertrophy (fig. 36)
3. True posterior (fig. 207) or lateral myocardial infarction
4. Wolff-Parkinson-White syndrome (fig. 152)
5. Left ventricular diastolic overloading
6. Muscular subaortic stenosis (fig. 228)
7. Duchenne dystrophy (25)

REFERENCES

BUNDLE-BRANCH BLOCK

1. DeForest, R. E.: Four cases of "benign" left bundle branch block in the same family. Am. Heart J. 1956: **51**, 398.
2. Evans, W., et al.: The significance of deep S waves in leads II and III. Brit. Heart J. 1960: **22**, 551.
3. Henry, E. I., et al.: Significance of the relation of QRS and T waves in bundle branch block: a useful electrocardiographic sign. Am. Heart J. 1957: **54**, 407.
4. Hiss, R. G., and Lamb, L. E.: Electrocardiographic findings in 122,043 individuals. Circulation 1962: **25**, 947.
5. Johnson, R. L., et al.: Electrocardiographic findings in 67,375 asymptomatic individuals. VI. Right bundle branch block. Am. J. Cardiol. 1960: **6**, 143.
6. Johnson, R. P., et al.: Prognosis in bundle branch block. II. Factors influencing the survival period in left bundle branch block. Am. Heart J. 1951: **41**, 225.
7. Lamb, L. E., et al.: Intermittent right bundle branch block without apparent heart disease. Am. J. Cardiol. 1959: **4**, 302.
8. Lamb, L. E., et al.: Electrocardiographic findings in 67,375 asymptomatic individuals. V. Left bundle branch block. Am. J. Cardiol. 1960: **6**, 130.
9. Lenegre, J.: Etiology and pathology of bilateral bundle branch block in relation to complete heart block. Progr. Cardiovasc. Dis. 1964: **6**, 409.
10. Lepeschkin, E.: The electrocardiographic diagnosis of bilateral bundle branch block in relation to heart block. Progr. Cardiovasc. Dis. 1964: **6**, 445.
11. Messer, A. L., et al.: Prognosis in bundle branch block. III. A comparison of right and left bundle branch block with a note on the relative incidence of each. Am. Heart J. 1951: **41**, 239.
12. Myers, G. B.: The form of the QRS complex in bundle branch block and in anterolateral infarction. Am. Heart J. 1950: **39**, 817.
13. Papp, C., and Smith, K. S.: The changing electrocardiogram in Wilson block. Circulation 1955: **11**, 53.
14. Scherf, D.: Intraventricular block. Am. J. Cardiol. 1960: **6**, 853.
15. Scott, R. C.: Left bundle branch block—a clinical assessment. Am. Heart J. 1965: **70**, 535, 691, and 813.
16. Shreenivas et al.: Prognosis in bundle branch block. I. Factors influencing the survival period in right bundle branch block. Am. Heart J. 1950: **40**, 891.
17. Sodi-Pallares, D.: *New Bases of Electrocardiography*. C. V. Mosby Co., St. Louis, 1956, pp. 289–292.
18. Tapia, F. A., and Proudfit, W. L.: Secondary R waves in right precordial leads in normal persons and in patients with cardiac disease. Circulation 1960: **21**, 28.

19. Unger, P. N., et al.: The concept of "masquerading" bundle-branch block: an electrocardiographic-pathologic correlation. Circulation 1958: **17,** 397.
20. Vazifdar, J. P., and Levine, S. A.: Benign bundle branch block. Arch. Int. Med. 1952: **89,** 568.
21. Wood, P.: Aortic stenosis. Am. J. Cardiol. 1958: **1,** 553.
22. deLeon, A. C., et al.: The straight back syndrome: clinical cardiovascular manifestations. Circulation 1965: **32,** 193.
23. DePasquale, N. P., and Burch, G. E.: Analysis of the RSR' complex in lead V_1. Circulation 1963: **28,** 362.

RATE-DEPENDENT BBB

24. Massumi, R. A.: Bradycardia-dependent bundle branch block. Circulation 1968: **38,** 1066.
25. Sarachek, N. S.: Bradycardia-dependent bundle branch block. Am. J. Cardiol. 1970: **25,** 727.

RSR' AND R PATTERNS IN RIGHT CHEST LEADS

26. Menendez, M. M., and Marriott, H. J. L.: Differential diagnosis of RSR' and dominant R wave patterns in right chest leads. J.A.M.A. 1966: **198,** 843.
27. Perloff, J. K., et al.: The cardiomyopathy of progressive muscular dystrophy. Circulation 1966: **33,** 625.
28. Chung, K. -Y., et al.: Wolff-Parkinson-White syndrome. Am. Heart J. 1965:**69,** 116.

8

The Hemiblocks and Trifascicular Block

In a series of fascinating publications, Rosenbaum (2–11) has established the concepts of "hemiblock" and "trifascicular block." Hemiblock is his term for blockage of one of the two main divisions of the left bundle branch.

The anterior division runs towards the base of the anterior papillary muscle of the left ventricle, the posterior division towards the posterior papillary muscle. Keep in mind that what anatomists have called anterior is really superior and posterior is really inferior (fig. 58). Activation of the left ventricle normally spreads simultaneously from these two locations— at the bases of the two papillary muscles. If the path to one of these is blocked, activation must begin exclusively from the other location; thus, if the anterior division is blocked (left anterior hemiblock or LAH), spread will begin at the base of the posterior papillary muscle and this will shift the general direction of spread upwards, from "posterior" to "anterior."

Because the posterior papillary muscle is situated not only below but also medial to the anterior muscle, the first activation is not only downwards but also somewhat rightward, and this initial spread will write a small Q in lead 1 with a small R in lead 3 (fig. 59); the remaining forces travel upwards and to the left to write an R in lead 1 and an S in lead 3 and so produce left axis deviation.

If the posterior division is blocked (left posterior hemiblock or LPH), activation will begin exclusively in the region of the anterior papillary muscle and the general direction of spread will be directed downwards and to the right. The first forces will travel upwards to the left (fig. 59) writing

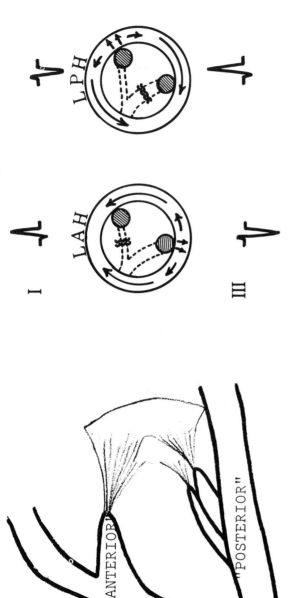

FIG. 59. Diagrams illustrating the hemiblock patterns in the limb leads: left anterior hemiblock (LAH) and left posterior hemiblock (LPH). The "anterior" papillary muscle is above and lateral to the "posterior" papillary muscle and the two divisions of the LBB course towards their respective papillary muscles. Thus, if the anterior division is blocked, initial electromotive forces are directed downwards and to the right, inscribing a Q wave in lead 1 and an R wave in lead 3. The subsequent forces are directed mainly upwards and to the left, writing an R wave in 1 and an S

(legend concluded opposite)

FIG. 58. The "anterior" papillary muscle of the left ventricle is above, rather than anterior to, the "posterior" papillary muscle.

in 2 and 3, to produce a left axis deviation. In LPH, the initial forces spread upwards and to the left to write an R in 1 and a Q in 3, while subsequent forces are directed downwards and to the right to produce right axis deviation. (Reproduced from Hemiblock Lecture Slides, Tampa Tracings, Oldsmar, Fla., 1971.)

a small R in lead 1 and small Q in lead 3. The remaining impulses, directed downwards and to the right, will write an S wave in lead 1 and an R wave in lead 3 and so shift the mean axis to the right.

Although the hemiblocks represent a form of intraventricular block, they do not lead to material widening of the QRS because the purkinje network in the territories of anterior and posterior divisions are richly confluent so that, although the order and direction of activation are dramatically changed, the time required for depolarization of the entire ventricle is barely increased—by 0.01–0.02 sec. at most.

The cardinal features of pure hemiblock are summarized in the box. Note that for LPH a fourth criterion is required: there must be no evidence of or reason for right ventricular hypertrophy. This additional criterion is necessary because right ventricular hypertrophy itself can produce exactly the same pattern as LPH.

Criteria for Left Anterior Hemiblock

1. Left axis deviation (usually −60°)
2. Small Q in lead 1, small R in 3
3. Normal QRS duration

Criteria for Left Posterior Hemiblock

1. Right axis deviation (usually +120°)
2. Small R in lead 1, small Q in 3
3. Normal QRS duration
4. No evidence for right ventricular hypertrophy

Although hemiblock can occur in pure form (fig. 60), LAH is often, and LPH almost always, associated with RBBB (figs. 61 and 62). In these cases the QRS complexes are of course abnormally wide because of the RBBB, not because of the hemiblock itself.

The hemiblocks have claim to some importance: first, LAH is much the most common cause of otherwise unexplained left axis deviation and, as such, fills a hitherto considerable gap in electrocardiographic knowledge. Second, both forms of hemiblock can play the alternate roles of mime and mask. LAH can *mimic* anterior infarction by producing Q waves in ante-

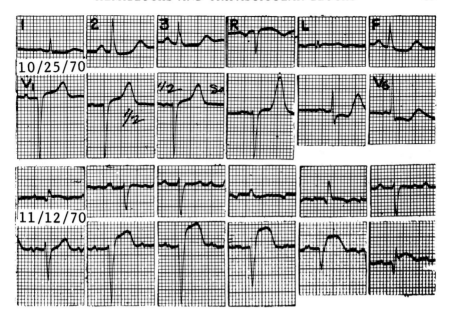

FIG. 60. **Left anterior hemiblock.** Between 10/25/70 and 11/12/70, definite evidence of acute anterior myocardial infarction has developed and the axis has swung "leftward" (superiorly) from +60° to −75°—definite evidence of LAH.

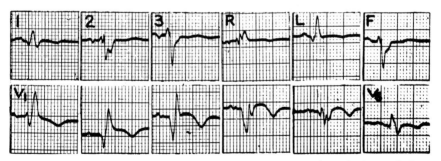

FIG. 61. **Right bundle-branch block + left anterior hemiblock** against a background of extensive anterior infarction.

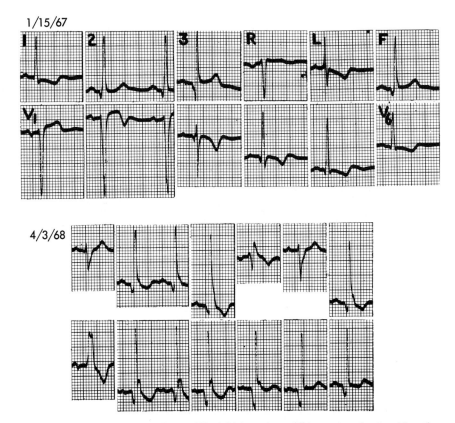

FIG. 62. **Left posterior hemiblock.** The initial tracing exhibits a normal axis with pathological Q waves in anterior (V$_{3-5}$) and inferior (2, 3 and aVF) leads. The later tracing illustrates widespread development of wide Q waves in the precordial leads with RBBB and
marked right axis deviation, presumably due to LPH. (Reproduced from Hemiblock Lecture
Slides, Tampa Tracings, Oldsmar, Fla., 1971.)

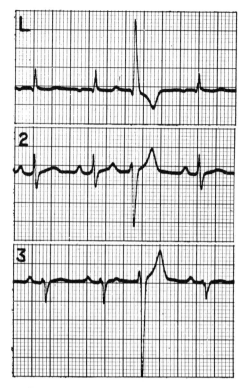

FIG. 63. Atrial premature beats with ventricular aberration of **left anterior hemiblock** type. In the aberrant beats, at the same time that the axis shifts markedly leftward to about −70°, the voltage of the QRS complexes greatly increases so that their pattern simulates that of left ventricular hypertrophy.

rior chest leads (especially if the electrodes are placed somewhat above the conventional level); lateral infarction by producing or enhancing Q waves in leads 1 and aVL; and left ventricular hypertrophy by increasing R-wave voltage in leads 1 and aVL (fig. 63). LAH can *mask* inferior infarction by substituting an R wave for a Q in leads 2, 3 and aVF (fig. 64); it can mask anteroseptal infarction (especially if the electrodes are placed somewhat below the conventional level) by converting a QS complex in anterior leads to an rS pattern; and left ventricular hypertrophy by diminishing R-wave voltage in left chest leads.

LPH can both mimic and mask anterior infarction. If the electrodes are placed somewhat below the conventional level, LPH can mimic infarction by producing Q waves in the anterior chest leads; and if the electrodes are placed somewhat above the conventional level, it can mask infarction by converting a QS complex into an rS pattern.

Left anterior hemiblock is common; left posterior hemiblock is rare. Several factors contribute to the relative immunity of the posterior division: first it is shorter and thicker than the anterior division; then it is an inflow-tract structure and thus avoids the stresses of outflow pressure and proximity to the danger area of the aortic valve; and thirdly, unlike the anterior division, it has a double blood supply.

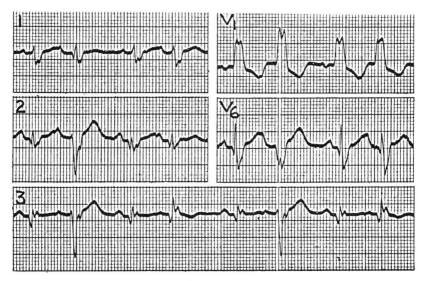

FIG. 64. Atrial bigeminy with RBBB and inferior infarction. The second beat in each lead, and the sixth beat in lead 3, show **left anterior hemiblock** aberration as well. In the limb leads, the development of LAH eliminates the Q waves in leads 2 and 3 and so masks the inferior infarction. (Reproduced from Hemiblock Lecture Slides, Tampa Tracings, Oldsmar, Fla. 1971.)

Hemiblock, like BBB, is commonly caused by ischemic heart disease and was found in 17 percent of 250 consecutive patients with acute myocardial infarction (1). Other causes include cardiomyopathy, Lev's disease, Lenegre's disease, and aortic valve calcification.

Miming and Masking by Hemiblocks		
	Can Mimic	Can Mask
LAH	Anterior infarction	Anterior infarction
	Lateral infarction	Inferior infarction
	Left ventricular	Left ventricular
	hypertrophy	hypertrophy
LPH	Anterior infarction	Anterior infarction.

TRIFASCICULAR BLOCK

Semantically, this term can be appropriately applied to simultaneous block, complete or incomplete, in any three of the five ventricular conducting fascicles (His bundle, RBB, LBB, anterior and posterior divisions of the LBB); but it is specifically applied to block simultaneously involving the three peripheral fascicles—the RBB and the two divisions of the LBB. Its manifestations are therefore varied and include all the eight possible combinations of complete and incomplete block in these three fascicles (see table). If all three fascicles are completely blocked, "complete A-V block" results. If the RBB and the anterior division block incompletely, the pattern of RBBB + left anterior hemiblock with "1st degree A-V block" appears; and so on.

The table lists the eight possible combinations with some of their electrocardiographic expressions. When incomplete block involves two or more fascicles, the number of possible variations is multiplied. For example, combination 8), with incomplete block in all three fascicles, could produce *any* of the expressions of trifascicular block, depending on the *relative* degree of incomplete block in each fascicle.

Manifestations of Trifascicular Block

	RBB	LAD	LPD	ECG Expression
1)	C	C	C	complete AVB
2)	C	C	I	RBBB + LAH + "AVB"
3)	C	I	C	RBBB + LPH + "AVB"
4)	I	C	C	LBBB + "AVB"
5)	C	I	I	various combinations
6)	I	C	I	depending upon relative
7)	I	I	C	degrees of incomplete
8)	I	I	I	fascicular block

Key: C = completely blocked
      I = incompletely blocked
      "AVB" = manifestations of 1st or 2nd degree A-V block

REFERENCES

1. Marriott, H. J. L., and Hogan, P.: Hemiblock in acute myocardial infarction. Chest 1970: **58,** 342.
2. Rosenbaum, M. B.: Types of right bundle branch block and their clinical significance. J. Electrocardiol. 1968: **1,** 221.
3. Rosenbaum, M. B.: Types of left bundle branch block and their clinical significance. J. Electrocardiol. 1969: **2,** 197.
4. Rosenbaum, M. B., et al.: Five cases of intermittent left anterior hemiblock. Am. J. Cardiol. 1969: **24,** 1.
5. Rosenbaum, M. B., et al.: The mechanism of bidirectional tachycardia. Am. Heart J. 1969: **78,** 4.
6. Rosenbaum, M. B., et al.: Intraventricular trifascicular blocks. The syndrome of right bundle branch block with intermittent left anterior and posterior hemiblock. Am. Heart J. 1969: **78,** 306.
7. Rosenbaum, M. B., et al.: Intraventricular trifascicular blocks. Review of the literature and classification. Am. Heart J. 1969: **78,** 450.
8. Rosenbaum, M. B.: The hemiblocks: diagnostic criteria and clinical significance. Mod. Conc. Cardiov. Dis. 1970: **39,** 141.
9. Rosenbaum, M. B., et al.: The hemiblocks: New concepts of intraventricular conduction based on human anatomical, physiological, and clinical studies. Tampa Tracings, Oldsmar, Fla., 1970.
10. Rosenbaum, M. B., et al.: Anatomical basis of AV conduction disturbances. Geriatrics 1970: **25,** 132.
11. Rosenbaum, M. B., et al.: Right bundle branch block with left anterior hemiblock surgically induced in tetralogy of Fallot. Am. J. Cardiol. 1970: **26,** 12.

9

And Now Arrhythmias

INTRODUCTION

Disturbances of rhythm are most conveniently divided into 1) supraventricular and 2) ventricular. This corresponds with a simple electrocardiographic difference—arrhythmias originating in the atrium or A-V junction (supraventricular), unless complicated by aberrant ventricular conduction (chapter 13), are characterized by normal QRS complexes, while ventricular arrhythmias produce bizarre QRST complexes with prolonged QRS interval.

With a prolonged interval there is always the possibility that abnormal intraventricular conduction is coincident with a supraventricular disturbance of rhythm. This may have been present before the supraventricular arrhythmia began, or the strain put upon ventricular conduction by an arrhythmic tachycardia may have induced a temporary intraventricular block. The pattern of abnormal intraventricular conduction plus supraventricular tachycardia may be virtually indistinguishable from ventricular tachycardia (see chapter 13).

Two other practical justifications for the subdivision of arrhythmias into supraventricular and ventricular are that 1) it is often impossible to distinguish between atrial and A-V tachycardias, and 2) the treatment of both supraventricular tachycardias is the same.

The diagnosis of an arrhythmia is often made at a glance. At other times, even the most painstaking and prolonged study is frustrated. In tracings requiring more than casual inspection it is well to approach the problem systematically. Since the QRS contains far more information that the P wave, and since the activity of the ventricles is of far greater concern than that of the atria, one should first *study the QRS complex:*

Is it normally narrow?   Indicating a supraventricular mechanism
Or is it widened?   If widened, apply all necessary available criteria to decide if it represents ectopic ventricular activity, or abnormal intraventricular conduction

Next, *identify P waves* and their site of origin (if necessary and possible). And finally, *establish relationships:*

Is the P related to the QRS?
Or are the ventricular complexes more consistently related to each other than to the P waves?
Or is the wave you think is a P wave constantly related to the preceding rather than to the following ventricular complex, as in figure 65?

Whenever you are faced with a defiant arrhythmia, be sure to keep these principles in mind.

Principles for Diagnosis

1. Milk the QRS
2. Cherchez le P
3. Who's married to whom?

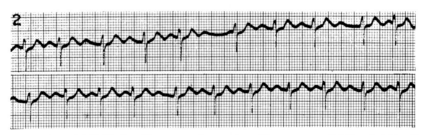

FIG. 65. **Atrial fibrillation.** Note unusually prominent U waves, superficially mimicking P waves.

Arrhythmias *may* be recognizable in any lead, but as a general rule V₁ is the best of the routine 12 leads: this is both because there are recognizable distinctions in this lead between the patterns of aberrant ventricular conduction and ectopic ventricular beats, and because it is the most likely to reveal skulking P waves. But it is folly to depend upon any single lead and, at times, it is necessary to search every lead available.

CONSTANT MONITORING

From chapter 7 it is evident that lead V₁ is an excellent, and usually the best, single lead for recognizing bundle-branch block patterns. Figure 40 illustrated the fact that bundle-branch block and ectopic ventricular impulses could produce remarkably similar complexes. And this is not surprising: bundle-branch block causes one ventricle to be activated ahead of the other and an ectopic impulse, beginning in one ventricle, has a similar effect. Thus bundle-branch block and ventricular ectopy cause the ventricles to be activated "in series" instead of "in parallel." If the *left* bundle branch is blocked, or if an ectopic impulse arises in the *right* ventricle, activation of the right ventricle will begin before the left; i.e., the general direction of activation will be from right to left. Since this general direction of spread is away from a right sided chest lead like V₁, LBBB and right ventricular ectopic beats will produce predominantly negative complexes in such a lead (see fig. 40). In contrast, RBBB and left ventricular ectopic beats will produce a predominantly left-to-right activation and will therefore inscribe mainly positive complexes in V₁ (fig. 66).

Lead V₁ is therefore the best single lead for distinguishing between right and left bundle branch block and between right and left ventricular ectopic

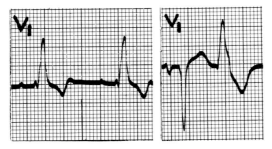

FIG. 66. The rsR′ pattern of RBBB (left) contrasted with the qR pattern of left ventricular ectopy (right).

beats. Even more important, as we shall see later (Chapter 13), V_1 is the best lead for distinguishing between left ventricular ectopic beats and ventricular aberration of RBBB type. Lead V_1 is also often the best lead for recording and recognizing atrial activity. Because V_1 possesses these several virtues, it would undoubtedly be the best of our 12 routine leads for the monitoring of patients for arrhythmias. But it is mechanically clumsy to keep a patient constantly attached to all four limb wires as well as the precordial wire. To obviate this mechanical difficulty and yet retain the diagnostic advantages of V_1, a modified bipolar chest lead ("MCL_1" = modified CL_1) was introduced and has served us well (1, 2).

The MCL_1 hook-up is illustrated in figure 67. The positive electrode is placed in the 4th right interspace (as for V_1) while the negative electrode is placed near the left shoulder usually under the outer third of the left clavicle. The ground wire is conveniently attached near the right shoulder.

Figure 68 illustrates RBBB, right and left ventricular premature beats, atrial premature beats with RBBB-type aberration, and a run of aberrant ventricular conduction of RBBB-type complicating atrial fibrillation. Many subsequent illustrations of the arrhythmias in this text will make use of this lead.

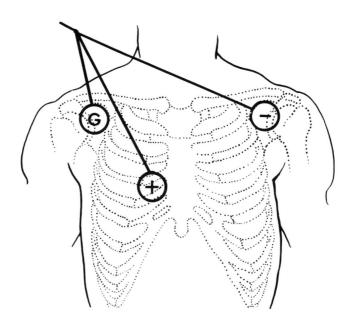

FIG. 67. Electrode placement of modified CL_1 (MCL_1).

ONE LEAD IS NOT ENOUGH

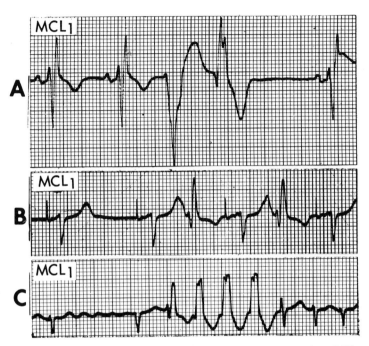

FIG. 68. Typical configurations in MCL₁: (A) Sinus beats show RBBB interrupted by right ventricular (rS) and left ventricular (qR) ectopic beats in succession. (B) Atrial pacing with two premature beats that have an rsR' contour and are preceded by P' waves—atrial premature beats with RBBB-type aberration. (C) Atrial fibrillation interrupted by a run of anomalous beats; the first has an rsR' pattern and indicates that the run is aberrant and not ectopic ventricular. (Reproduced from Marriott and Fogg, Constant monitoring for cardiac dysrhythmias and blocks. Mod. Conc. Cardiovasc. Dis. 1970: **39,** 103; by permission of the American Heart Assoc.)

REFERENCES

1. Marriott, H. J. L., and Fogg, E.: Constant monitoring for arrhythmias and blocks. Mod. Conc. Cardiovasc. Dis. 1970: **39,** 103.
2. Marriott, H. J. L., and Thorne, D. C.: Dysrhythmic dilemmas in coronary care. Am. J. Cardiol. 1971: 27, 327.

GLOSSARY

Aberrant ventricular conduction. The temporarily abnormal intraventricular conduction of a supraventricular impulse, usually associated with a change in cycle length.

Accelerated idionodal rhythm. An automatic A-V rhythm, controlling only the ventricles, at a rate between 60 and 100 beats per minute.

Accelerated idioventricular rhythm. An automatic ectopic ventricular rhythm, controlling only the ventricles, at a rate between 50 and 100 beats per minute.

Atrial capture. Conduction to the atria, from A-V junction or ventricles, after a period of A-V dissociation.

Automaticity. The property inherent in all pacemaking cells that enables them to form new impulses spontaneously.

Automatic beat or **rhythm.** A beat or rhythm arising in a spontaneously beating center, independent of the dominant sinus (or other) rhythm.

A-V dissociation. Independent beating of atria and ventricles.

Block. Pathological delay or interruption of impulse conduction.

Bradycardia. Any heart (or chamber) rhythm having an average rate under 60 beats per minute.

Capture(d) beat. A conducted beat following a period of A-V dissociation.

Concealed conduction. Conduction of an impulse within the A-V junction, recognizable only by its effect on the subsequent beat or cycle.

Coupling interval. The interval between an extrasystole and the beat preceding it.

Ectopic beat. A beat arising in any focus other than the sinus node.

Ectopy. Ectopic impulse formation.

Escape(d) beat. An automatic beat ending a cycle longer than the dominant cycle and able to appear only because of a slowing or interruption of the dominant rhythm.

Extrasystole. An ectopic beat, dependent upon and coupled to the preceding beat.

Fusion beat. A beat resulting from the simultaneous spread of more than one impulse through the same myocardial territory (either ventricles or atria).

Idionodal rhythm. An independent rhythm arising in the A-V junction and controlling only the ventricles.

Idioventricular rhythm. A rhythm arising in and controlling only the ventricles.

Isorhythmic dissociation. A-V dissociation during which atria and ventricles are beating at the same or almost the same rate.

Parasystole. An automatic ectopic rhythm whose pacemaker is "protected" from discharge by the sinus or other circumnavigating impulses so that it is able to maintain its own uninterrupted rhythm in competition with the dominant rhythm.

Premature beat. An ectopic beat, dependent upon and coupled to the preceding beat, and occurring before the next expected dominant beat.

Tachyarrhythmia. Any disturbance of rhythm resulting in a heart or chamber rate over 100 beats per minute.

Tachycardia. Any heart (or chamber) rhythm having an average rate over 100 beats per minute.

Ventricular aberration. Aberrant ventricular conduction.

Ventricular capture. Conduction to the ventricles after a period of A-V dissociation.

Wolff-Parkinson-White syndrome. An electrocardiographic "syndrome" consisting of a short P-R interval (<0.12 sec.) with widened QRS complex including a delta wave (slurred initial component).

10

Ventricular Arrhythmias

VENTRICULAR PREMATURE BEATS

The terms **ectopic beat, premature beat** and **extrasystole** are in usage virtually synonymous. Not all ectopic beats, however, are premature. For example the ventricular escape beat is ectopic but, by definition, far from being premature, it is *late;* and it is important not to confuse it with the sometimes dastardly premature beat, because the escape beat is indeed a friend in need. And again, the ventricular response in atrial fibrillation may be interrupted by an ectopic ventricular beat; but as the time of the next ventricular response during atrial fibrillation usually cannot be predicted, it is ridiculous to call such a beat premature.

The isolated ventricular premature beat (VPB) is an easily spotted anomaly—it sticks out grotesquely like a sore thumb. Several are shown in figures 69 to 77. The ectopic impulses produce distorted QRST complexes, all of which have certain characteristics in common: 1) they anticipate the next normal impulse (i.e., they are premature); 2) the QRS intervals are prolonged; 3) the ST segments slope away in the direction opposite to the main QRS deflections; 4) following each premature beat there is a relatively long pause before the next sinus impulse in due time initiates the next cardiac cycle; this pause "compensates" for the prematurity of the ectopic beat so that the interval from the beat preceding the ectopic beat to that following it is exactly equal to two cardiac cycles: e.g., in strip A in figure 70 the interval from b to c equals that from a to b. The pause following the premature beat is therefore **fully compensatory** in contrast with the interval that follows a supraventricular beat (strip B in fig. 70). In strip B the interval from b to c is shorter than a to b. However, the compensatory

102

pause as a diagnostic prop is something of a broken reed and several exceptions to these principles will be noted.

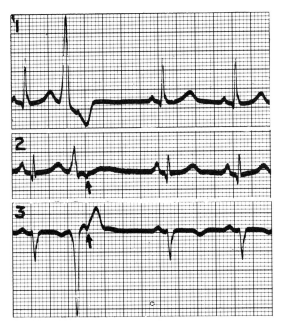

FIG. 69. **Ventricular premature beats.** The second beat in each lead is a ventricular premature beat. Incidentally, they show retrograde conduction to the atria (retrograde P waves—arrow), a common phenomenon.

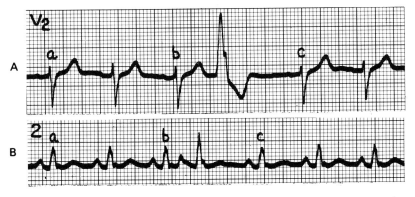

FIG. 70. Comparison of interval following **ventricular premature beat** (A) and that following an **atrial premature beat** (B); see text.

The P wave is usually lost in the VPB because the QRS complex is usually early enough to swamp it. Occasionally it may be seen as a notch or splinter slightly deforming some part of the QRS complex, ST segment or the T wave (fig. 71 A). On the other hand, if the ectopic beat is only slightly premature, the normal P wave may have time to put in an appearance shortly before the abnormal QRS (fig. 71 B) and the extrasystole is then called "end-diastolic." Occasionally the ectopic beat is so premature that the next sinus impulse finds the ventricle sufficiently recovered to respond. In such circumstances the premature beat is sandwiched in between two consecutive sinus beats and is known as an **interpolated beat** (fig. 72 B).

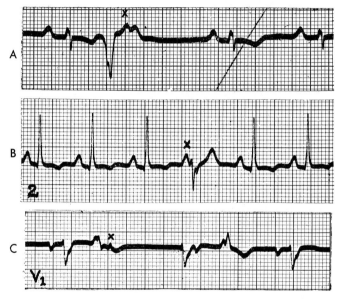

FIG. 71. Relationship of P waves to **ventricular premature beats.** In A the ventricular beat is very premature and the P wave (x) deforms the ST segment. In B the ectopic beat is only slightly premature and the P wave (x) precedes it. In C the first premature beat is followed by a retrograde P wave (x); retrograde conduction to the atria is not observed following the second premature beat.

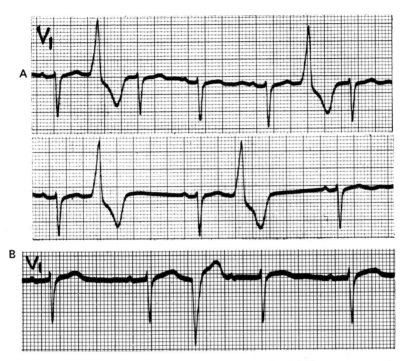

FIG. 72. **Ventricular premature beats.** In the upper strip of A the two extrasystoles are interpolated; in the lower strip each is followed by a fully compensatory pause. In B, the VPB is interpolated with concealed retroconduction prolonging the ensuing P-R interval.

The ectopic impulse from the ventricles often spreads backwards into the atria, inscribing a retrograde P wave which replaces the sinus P wave that was otherwise expected (5) (figs. 69 and 71 C). Sometimes the retrograde impulse enters the A-V junction but fails to reach the atria; in such circumstances, penetration into the A-V junction may leave the tissues refractory so that the next descending sinus impulse is delayed and a long P-R interval produced (fig. 72 B). This is why the sinus beat following an interpolated ventricular premature beat often has a prolonged P-R interval. Because the conduction backwards into the A-V tissues is recognizable only by its effect on the subsequent beat, it is known as **concealed retrograde conduction** (8).

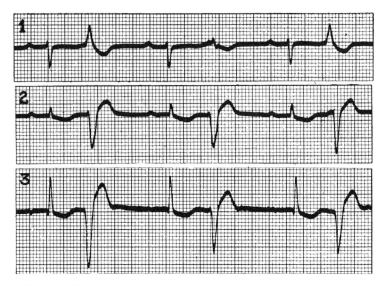

FIG. 73. **Bigeminal rhythm.** In each lead every alternate beat is a ventricular premature beat. In this patient the extrasystoles were due to digitalis intoxication, and their pattern is characteristically not uniform.

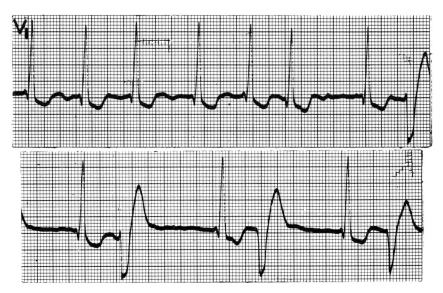

FIG. 74. The "**rule of bigeminy**" in action during atrial fibrillation. Abrupt lengthening of the ventricular cycle towards the end of the top strip precipitates a ventricular premature beat; the relatively long cycle following each successive VPB precipitates another—and so bigeminy tends to be self-perpetuating.

When every other beat is a premature beat (fig. 73) the rhythm is described as **bigeminy (pulsus bigeminus, bigeminal rhythm)** or **coupling**. By the "rule of bigeminy" (9), bigeminal rhythm tends to be self-perpetuating. This is because a long cycle tends to precipitate a ventricular premature beat (fig. 74); and so, once one premature beat has been produced, the lengthened postextrasystolic cycle tends to produce another—and so on and on. If every third beat is a premature beat (fig. 75 A), or if each normal beat is followed by a pair of premature beats (fig. 75 B and C), **trigeminy (pulsus trigeminus, trigeminal rhythm)** is produced. Trigeminy can

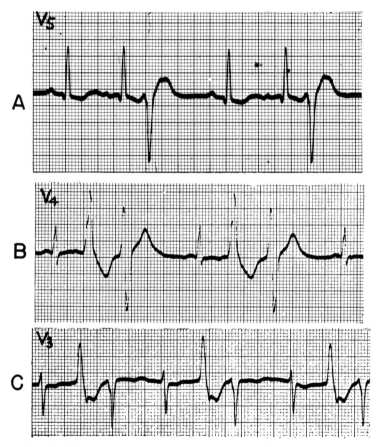

FIG. 75. **Trigeminal rhythm,** two forms. In A every third beat is a ventricular premature beat; in B and C each sinus beat is followed by a pair of ventricular premature beats.

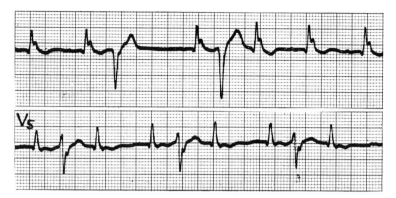

FIG. 76. **Trigeminal rhythm.** In the upper strip the first ectopic beat is followed by a compensatory pause; the second, being slightly more premature, is interpolated. In the bottom strip every third beat is an interpolated extrasystole, with the result that the heart beats occur in groups of three (trigeminy).

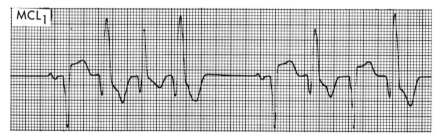

FIG. 77. **Ventricular quadrigeminy.** The first quartet is composed of one sinus beat followed by three left ventricular premature beats. The second foursome consists of a sinus beat followed by an interpolated VPB, another sinus beat and another VPB.

also be produced by interpolated extrasystoles occurring every third beat (fig. 76). And when such a trigeminal group is followed by another premature beat (fig. 77), the quadruplet so formed is one type of quadrigeminy; another results when three consecutive premature beats follow the sinus beat (fig. 77).

It is well known that premature beats with short coupling intervals are more likely to precipitate a dangerous ventricular tachyarrhythmia (fig. 78). The danger zone (vulnerable period) corresponds roughly with the peak of the T wave, and if a premature beat lands on the preceding T wave (R-on-T phenomenon), it may spark ventricular tachycardia or fibrillation (24). The acutely damaged myocardium is especially susceptible to this disaster, to which any coronary care crew will testify.

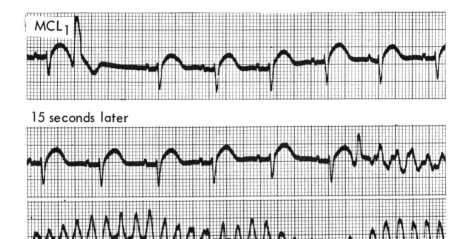

FIG. 78. **Ventricular fibrillation.** The second beat in the top strip is an early left ventricular premature beat. Towards the end of the second strip, the R-on-T phenomenon precipitates ventricular fibrillation. (From a 50-year-old nurse who returned to full time work.)

Ectopic ventricular beats are generally regarded as a normal finding unless they are very numerous or arise from more than one focus (**multifocal or multiform ectopic beats**) (fig. 75 B and C). Even bigeminal rhythm, however, is sometimes seen in an otherwise normal heart. When both ventricular and atrial ectopic beats are observed in the same heart, it is often considered evidence of cardiac disease (22).

MORPHOLOGY OF ECTOPIC VENTRICULAR BEATS

The introduction of constant monitoring, especially in coronary care units, has highlighted the need to distinguish between ectopic ventricular rhythms and supraventricular rhythms with intraventricular conduction disturbances. It has also given us the opportunity to study the problem intensively and this in turn has led to the recognition of certain clues of great value in making this distinction (13, 16).

The most important of these clues has been in the details of QRS morphology. After monitoring several hundred patients with a right chest lead (MCL$_1$), nurses in the Coronary Care Center at St. Anthony's hospital observed that left ventricular ectopic complexes tended to peak *early;* their upstroke was steep whereas their downstroke was slurred, or, if they formed two distinct peaks (fig. 79), the left "rabbit-ear" was taller than the right. A count of left ventricular extrasystoles then showed that this was true of about half such beats, whereas about a quarter of left ventricular beats peaked late. This has proved of great differential value because it is most uncommon for RBBB aberration to present an early peak, i.e., "left rabbit-ear taller than right."

Corresponding complexes in V_6 or MCL_6 present an rS or QS complex and almost never have a small initial Q wave (fig. 79); whereas most aberrant beats of RBBB-type present a qRs configuration. Figure 80 shows a good example of a ventricular tachycardia illustrating the classical features of left ventricular ectopy in V_1 and V_6.

Two other clues that seem to be of significant value:

1) The presence of concordant complexes all across the precordium, i.e., all negative or all positive (12, 14). If they are all positive it is almost certainly ectopic ventricular provided a W-P-W syndrome can be excluded; and if they are all negative, it is almost certainly ectopic, the only exception being an occasional example of LBBB in which an upright complex is not yet obtained in V_6 but is obtainable at V_7.

2) An axis in the frontal plane between -90 and -180 degrees (fig. 80).

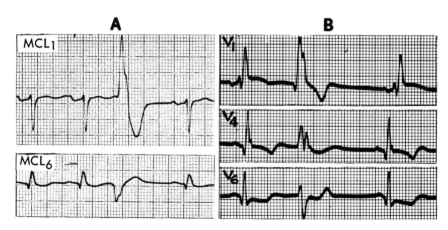

Fig. 79. **Left ventricular premature beats.** Two characteristic precordial forms: In A, a qR in MCL_1 (with steep upstroke to an early peak and slurred downstroke) and QS in MCL_6; in B, qR in V_1 (with left "rabbit-ear" taller than right) with rS in V_6. Compare classic morphology of RBBB in flanking sinus beats.

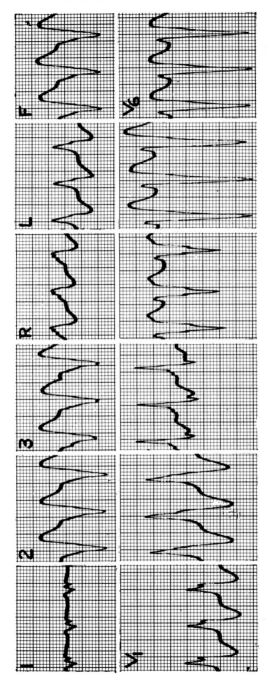

FIG. 80. **Ventricular tachycardia.** Note monophasic R in V_1 with left "rabbit-ear" taller than right, rS pattern in V_6, and bizarre frontal plane axis ($-100°$).

> ### Salient Features of Ventricular Premature Beats
>
> 1. Bizarre, premature QRST complex, with prolonged QRS interval and ST segment sloping off in direction opposite to main QRS deflection
> 2. Morphological details sometimes characteristic
> 3. Followed by *fully* compensatory pause (unless interpolated)
> 4. P wave usually lost (submerged in ventricular complex), sometimes retrograde

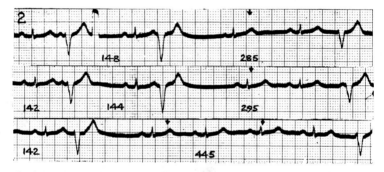

FIG. 81. **Ventricular parasystole.** The strips are continuous. Note the ectopic beats with varying coupling intervals. The inter-ectopic intervals are noted at the bottom of each strip (in hundredths of a second). Note that the shortest inter-ectopic intervals range from 142 to 148; the longer intervals are approximate multiples (285 = 2 × 142; 295 = 2 × 147; 445 = 3 × 148). The small arrows at the top of each strip indicate where the parasystolic center discharged but found the ventricles refractory.

VENTRICULAR PARASYSTOLE

Ventricular premature beats tend to occur during the supernormal recovery phase of the ventricle which corresponds with the U wave in the electrocardiogram. During this phase of supernormal excitability the ventricles can be activated by stimuli which are otherwise sub-threshold. Premature beats therefore tend to bear a fixed relationship to the preceding beat; this fixed relationship is known as **fixed coupling,** and the ectopic beat is thought to be in some way causally related to—"forced by", "dependent upon"—the preceding beat.

Sometimes, however, an autonomous ectopic focus in the ventricle fires off regular impulses at its own independent rate, and whenever these impulses arise at a time outside the refractory period, an ectopic beat results. This phenomenon of a parallel pacemaker competing for control is known as **parasystole** and it is able to maintain its own independent rhythm because it is in some way "protected" from being discharged by outside impulses. Parasystole is to be suspected whenever 1) the ectopic beats show a varying time relationship to the preceding beats (**variable coupling**) and 2) the intervals between consecutive ectopic beats are all equal to or are multiples of the shortest inter-ectopic interval observed (fig. 81). It is possible that in some cases the slow manifest parasystolic discharge in reality masks an underlying ventricular tachycardia (20, 22).

VENTRICULAR FUSION BEATS

Fusion beats—also known as summation or combination beats—result when the ventricles are partly activated by a descending atrial impulse and partly by an ectopic ventricular focus. Such beats are seen when extrasystoles occur late in diastole (fig. 82), and in parasystole when the parasys-

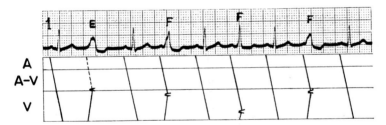

FIG. 82. **Ventricular fusion beats.** Fusion occurs on three occasions (F) between the sinus impulse and an ectopic ventricular impulse. The ectopic beats are producing a bigeminal rhythm, they occur late in diastole, and their coupling interval to the preceding sinus beat varies. The diagram below the tracing illustrates the varying levels of fusion in the three beats (F). The second beat in the strip (E) is a fullblown ectopic beat. The first fusion beat looks more like the ectopic pattern than a sinus beat and is obviously composed mainly of ectopic spread with only a minor contribution from the descending sinus impulse. The second fusion beat looks more like a sinus beat and clearly owes most to the sinus impulse. The third fusion beat is almost all ectopic but is just different enough in contour from the ectopic beat to be sure that the sinus impulse contributed slightly to its pattern.

tolic impulse happens to coincide with a sinus beat (fig. 83). Fusion beats are also commonly seen in accelerated idioventricular rhythms (see pp. 116–119) and when the heart is being artificially paced (see chapter 17). Fixed rate pacemakers (producing as they do an artificial ventricular parasystole) and demand pacemakers (which produce an artificial ventricular escape) are potent manufacturers of fusion beats. Each of two impulses, entering the ventricular myocardium more or less simultaneously, activates a variable portion of the ventricles, producing QRS-T complexes that are intermediate in form and duration between the sinus beats and the ectopic beats. Fusion beats interrupting ventricular tachycardia are often called Dressler beats (3).

There are two exceptional situations in which two impulses, each of which alone produces a wide, abnormal QRS complex, conspire to write a narrow, normal-looking fusion complex. If, in the presence of complete A-V block, two idioventricular pacemakers, one in each ventricle, discharge their impulses more or less simultaneously, both ventricles are activated at the same time and the resulting QRS complex may look entirely normal (fig. 84). Similarly, if in the presence of BBB, an ectopic ventricular center

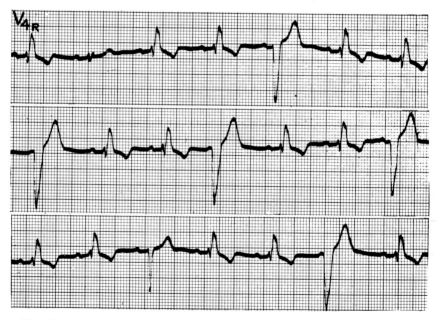

FIG. 83. **Ventricular fusion beats.** Sinus rhythm with RBBB punctuated by regularly occurring right ventricular ectopic beats (parasystole). The 2nd and 5th beats in top strip and 3rd beat in bottom strip are fusion beats. That in the bottom strip illustrates how two impulses—each of which individually creates a wide QRS complex—can produce a normally narrow fusion complex.

on the same side as the block discharges at the same instant that the descending sinus impulse enters the other ventricle, again both are activated simultaneously to write a narrow complex (figs. 83 and 85).

Fusion beats are of considerable importance in diagnosis. For fusion to occur, at least one of the fusing impulses presumably must arise within the

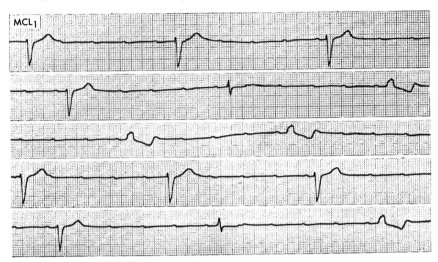

FIG. 84. **Complete A-V block** with two competing idioventricular pacemakers, one in each ventricle (right ventricular in 1st and 4th strips, left ventricular in 3rd strip). In the 2nd and 5th strips, the middle beats are narrow fusion beats thanks to simultaneous activation of the two ventricles.

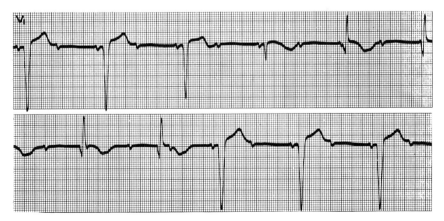

FIG. 85. **Ventricular fusion beats.** Two sinus beats with LBBB are followed by 2 or 3 fusion beats and then pure left idioventricular beats. The 4th beat in the top strip is normally narrow since the sinus impulse is activating the right ventricle while the ectopic ventricular impulse is simultaneously activating the left.

ventricles, since it is inconceivable that both of two supraventricular impulses, competing for the "final common path" of the His bundle, can enter the ventricles and fuse within them. Therefore, the argument runs, if fusion beats can be demonstrated there must be a ventricular focus at work.

Unfortunately, this does not completely hold water, and it *is* possible for fusion to occur between two supraventricular impulses if one of them descends by orthodox paths while the other arises in the A-V junction and travels by "paraspecific" fibers so that it enters the ventricles by a "side door" and spreads aberrantly (7). And of course in many W-P-W syndromes *every* beat represents fusion between two supraventricular impulses. Nevertheless, in most circumstances, the demonstration of fusion is regarded as good circumstantial evidence of ventricular ectopy.

ACCELERATED IDIOVENTRICULAR RHYTHMS

Before the coronary care era, this group of rhythm disturbances received virtually no attention. With the advent of constant monitoring, it has become clear that ectopic ventricular rhythms at rates under 100 are about as common after myocardial infarction as is ventricular tachycardia, occurring in about 20 per cent of cases. Characterized by a ventricular rate between 50 and 100, they have been lumped together under a variety of inappropriate (nonparoxysmal ventricular tachycardia (19), idioventricular tachycardia (21)), and even ridiculous (slow ventricular tachycardia (1)) names. Until they are better understood, I prefer to call them **accelerated (idio)ventricular rhythms.**

Disturbances of rhythm that qualify for this category often have a rate similar to the prevailing sinus rate and owe their appearance to slight slowing of the sinus pacemaker or to slight acceleration by the ectopic center. They therefore frequently begin with a fusion beat or two (fig. 86), produce a short run of isorhythmic dissociation (17), and then yield control to the sinus pacemaker again. In some instances, instead of dissociation

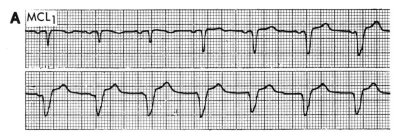

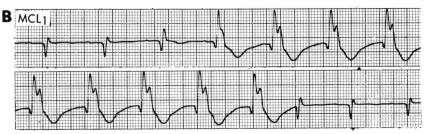

FIG. 86. **Accelerated idioventricular rhythm.** A. From the right ventricle—the 4th, 5th and 6th beats in the top strip are fusion beats. B. From the left ventricle. Note the left "rabbit-ear" taller than the right. In the top strip the 3rd and 4th beats are fusion beats.

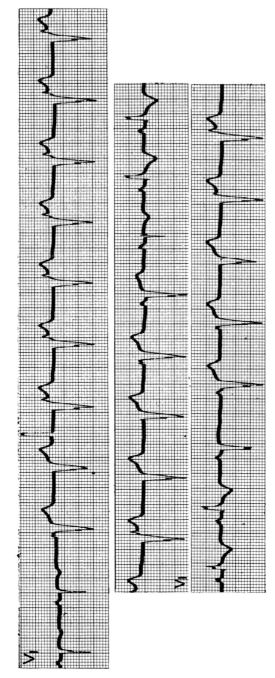

FIG. 87. **Accelerated ventricular rhythm.** In top strip, the first two beats *appear to be* normally conducted sinus beats. The sinus rhythm then slows and permits an ectopic right ventricular pacemaker to escape at an almost identical rate. The first two ectopic beats are dissociated from the sinus rhythm, but after that retrograde conduction to the atria develops (narrow positive spike deforming early part of ST segments) and continues to end of strip.

Bottom two strips are continuous and begin with the accelerated ventricular rhythm with retroconduction in its first beat; then come three dissociated beats, then two fusion beats, the second of which looks like a normally conducted sinus beat. Four sinus beats follow with incomplete RBBB and then a return to the accelerated ventricular rhythm via a fusion beat with retroconduction again in the two final beats.

Now we can recognize the identity of the first two beats in the top strip and the 6th beat in the 2nd strip—they look like normal beats because they represent fusion between a right ventricular impulse and a sinus impulse conducted with RBBB (p. 114).

between the two pacemakers, there is retrograde conduction to the atria (fig. 87). Some of these rhythms are parasystolic but the majority are not; some runs begin with an early ectopic beat, though most begin with an end-diastolic fusion beat; some show variation in rate, though most are constant and regular. It is clear that this term embraces a group of disorders of ventricular rhythm, not a single mechanism. The most important thing to know about them is that they are generally benign and do not as a rule lead to more dangerous arrhythmias.

VENTRICULAR PAROXYSMAL TACHYCARDIA

Ventricular tachycardia (VT) can be thought of as a run of rapidly repeated premature beats. It therefore consists of at least three consecutive, bizarre, prolonged QRS complexes recurring at a rapid rate. They are usually regular, despite the widespread doctrine that irregularity helps to identify ventricular tachycardia. One of the reasons for this popular belief is that so many examples of atrial fibrillation with W-P-W conduction have been mistakenly published as VT (15). The P waves are frequently lost in the barrage of ventricular complexes, though they may sometimes be recognized as notches occurring at a slower rate and usually in no constant relationship to the ventricular complexes (figs. 88, 89, and 90 A). Identification of unrelated P waves is one of the most sought after clues in recognizing ventricular tachycardia; yet atrial independence by no means proves a ventricular origin—it just excludes an atrial origin.

** YOU CANNOT TELL A PACEMAKER BY THE COMPANY SHE DOESN'T KEEP **

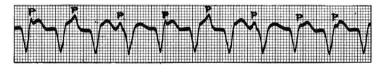

FIG. 88. **Ventricular tachycardia** at relatively slow rate of 120. Independent P waves are seen at slower rate (92).

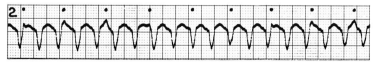

FIG. 89. **Ventricular tachycardia** at rate 200. Independent atrial activity is indicated by the superposed dots.

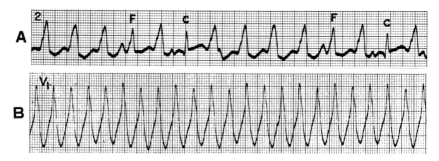

FIG. 90. **Ventricular tachycardia.** A. Relatively slow ventricular rate (126), with obvious large independent P waves. On two occasions (C) the atrial impulse completely captures the ventricles, while on two others (F) it only partially captures, to result in a fusion (Dressler) beat. B. Typical pattern of rapid ventricular tachycardia, rate 204; atrial activity is not discernible.

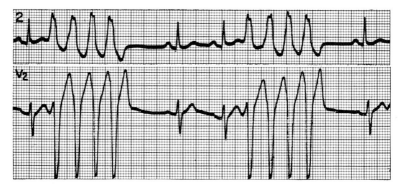

FIG. 91. Short 4-beat bursts of **ventricular tachycardia**

Ventricular tachycardia sometimes occurs in short repeated bursts, separated by one or two sinus beats (fig. 91), and then is known as **repetitive tachycardia** (25). It is often impossible to differentiate true ventricular tachycardia from a supraventricular tachycardia complicated by intraventricular block. The combination of supraventricular tachycardia with intraventricular block may be suspected, however, if the patient is known to have been subject to supraventricular arrhythmias, i.e., if atrial premature beats or atrial tachycardia, for example, have been observed in previous tracings. It may be strongly suspected if the patient had a pre-existing bundle-branch block, and with the onset of the tachycardia the pattern of the QRST complexes appears unchanged; or if the morphological patterns typical of aberrant ventricular conduction are present (see chapter 13); or if abnormal P waves are seen in constant relationship to each abnormal QRS complex. Even in these circumstances the possibility of a ventricular

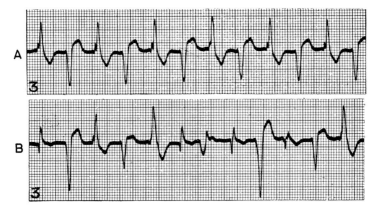

FIG. 92. Two serious forms of ventricular tachycardia, often presaging ventricular fibrillation. A. **Bidirectional ventricular tachycardia.** B. **Multifocal ventricular tachycardia** (sometimes called **chaotic heart action**).

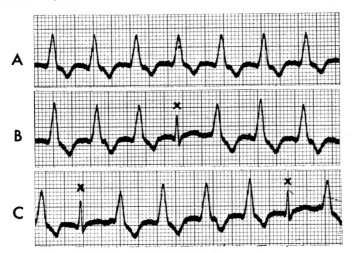

FIG. 93. **Ventricular tachycardia.** A. Typical form at relatively slow rate of 130. B and C form a continuous strip in which occasional atrial impulses are conducted (x).

tachycardia with retrograde conduction to the atria can usually not be excluded—and such retrograde conduction is quite common (6).

Another pattern almost diagnostic of ventricular tachycardia is shown in figures 90A, 93 where a suspected ventricular tachycardia is punctuated by an occasional fusion (Dressler) beat (3). These are sometimes to be seen when the ventricular rate is relatively slow and indicate that an impulse from the independently beating atria, happening to arrive at an opportune moment when the ventricles were no longer refractory, has been partially conducted. To fulfill the necessary criteria, such beats must be on time or slightly early, never late.

Another useful pointer to ventricular tachycardia is the presence of early ventricular capture beats that show a more normal QRS contour than the wide beats of the tachycardia (fig. 94). Since the capture beat ends a cycle slightly shorter than the cycles ending with the wider beats, it indicates that the wider beats are probably ectopic ventricular. Because, of all the beats, the *most likely* to be aberrant is the beat that ends the shortest cycle. Since this beat is not aberrant, the wide beats are even less likely to be and are therefore wide and bizarre because of ventricular ectopy rather than aberration.

And finally, of course, the same details of QRS morphology, outlined earlier in this chapter for the recognition of ventricular premature beats, are of equal importance in the recognition of ventricular tachycardia. Further details of the differential diagnosis of ventricular tachycardia are discussed in chapter 13.

Ventricular tachycardia is less common than atrial tachycardia, but it is much more serious. It is usually a sign of grave heart disease and is a not uncommon prelude to ventricular fibrillation. **Ventricular flutter** is the term given by some authorities to a rapid ventricular tachycardia giving a modified pattern in the electrocardiogram—a regular zigzag, without clearly formed QRS complexes (fig. 95 B and C). Nothing is gained in separating it from ventricular tachycardia.

Ventricular fibrillation is usually a terminal, or at least a catastrophic, event; rarely, transient bouts may be responsible for Adams-Stokes at-

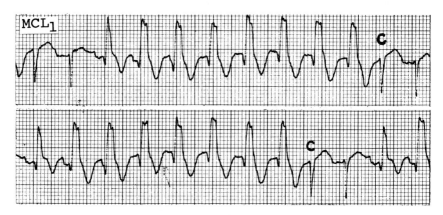

FIG. 94. **Ventricular tachycardia.** The capture beats (c) end cycles that are slightly shorter than the ectopic cycles. Note also: each run of ectopic rhythm begins with a fusion beat and the left "rabbit-ear" is taller than the right.

tacks. It is easily recognized by the complete absence of properly formed
ventricular complexes—the baseline wavers unevenly with no attempt at
forming clearcut QRS deflections (fig. 95 E and F).

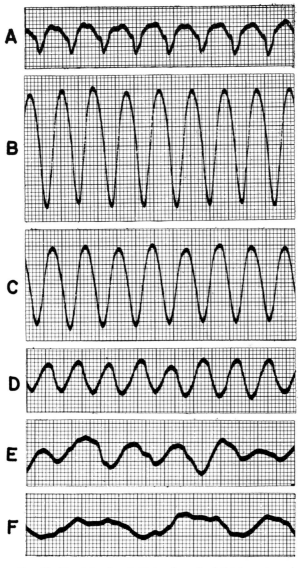

FIG. 95. **The dying heart.** Strips from lead 2 taken approximately 1 min. apart and illustrating the transitions from ventricular tachycardia through flutter to fibrillation. A. **Ventricular
tachycardia.** B and C. **Ventricular flutter.** D. Intermediate stage
between flutter and fibrillation. E and F. **Ventricular fibrillation.**

REFERENCES

1. Castellanos, A. et al.: Mechanisms of slow ventricular tachycardias in acute myocardial infarction. Dis. Chest 1969: **56,** 470.
2. Cohn, L. J., et al.: Ventricular tachycardia. Progr. Cardiovasc. Dis. 1966: **9,** 29.
3. Dressler, W., and Roesler, H.: The occurrence in paroxysmal ventricular tachycardia of ventricular complexes transitional in shape to sinoauricular beats. Am. Heart J. 1952: **44,** 485.
4. Huppert, V. F., and Berliner, K.: Auricular premature systoles occurring at rapid heart rates. Bull. N. Y. Med. Coll. 1951: **14,** 23.
5. Kistin, A., and Landowne, M.: Retrograde conduction from premature ventricular contractions, a common occurrence in the human heart. Circulation 1951: **3,** 738.
6. Kistin, A. D.: Retrograde conduction to the atria in ventricular tachycardia. Circulation 1961: **24,** 236.
7. Kistin, A. D.: Problems in the differentiation of ventricular arrhythmia from supraventricular arrhythmia with abnormal QRS. Progr. Cardiovasc. Dis. 1966: **9,** 1.
8. Langendorf, R.: Concealed A-V conduction. Am. Heart J. 1948: **35,** 542.
9. Langendorf, R. et al.: Mechanisms of intermittent ventricular bigeminy. I. Appearance of ectopic beats dependent upon the length of the ventricular cycle, the "rule of bigeminy". Circulation 1955: **11,** 422.
10. Mack, I., and Langendorf, R.: Factors influencing the time of appearance of premature systoles. Circulation 1950: **1,** 910.
11. Marriott, H. J. L., et al.: Ventricular fusion beats. Circulation 1962: **26,** 880.
12. Marriott, H. J. L.: Differential diagnosis of supraventricular and ventricular tachycardia. Geriatrics 1970: **25,** 91.
13. Marriott, H. J. L., and Fogg, E.: Constant monitoring for arrhythmias and blocks. Mod. Conc. Cardiovasc. Dis. 1970: **39,** 103.
14. Marriott, H. J. L., and Myerburg, R. J.: in Hurst and Logue, *The Heart*, ed. 2, McGraw Hill, New York, 1970, pp. 513–514.
15. Marriott, H. J. L., and Rogers, H. M.: Mimics of ventricular tachycardia associated with the W-P-W syndrome. J. Electrocardiol. 1969: **2,** 77.
16. Marriott, H. J. L., and Thorne, D. C.: Dysrhythmic dilemmas in coronary care. Am. J. Cardiol. 1971: **27,** 327.
17. Massumi, R. A., and Ali, N.: Accelerated isorhythmic ventricular rhythms. Am. J. Cardiol. 1970: **26,** 170.
18. Pick, A.: Parasystole. Circulation 1953: **8,** 243.
19. Rothfeld, E. L., et al.: Nonparoxysmal ventricular tachycardia. Circulation 1967: **36** (supp. 2), 227.
20. Schamroth, L.: Ventricular parasystole with slow manifest ectopic discharge. Brit. Heart J. 1962: **24,** 731.
21. Schamroth, L. Idioventricular tachycardia. J. Electrocardiol. 1968: **1,** 205.
22. Scherf, D., and Schott, A.: *Extrasystoles and Allied Arrhythmias*. Grune and Stratton, New York, 1953.
23. Scherf, D., and Bornemann, C.: Parasystole with a rapid ventricular center. Am. Heart J. 1961: **62,** 320.
24. Smirk, F. H., and Palmer, D. G.: A myocardial syndrome, with particular reference to the occurrence of sudden death and of premature systoles interrupting antecedent T waves. Am. J. Cardiol. 1960: **6,** 620.
25. Stock, J. P. P.: Repetitive paroxysmal ventricular tachycardia. Brit. Heart J. 1962: **24,** 297.

More Practical Points

The technician is not expected to learn how to interpret the tracing, but she should be told certain useful points that will make her work more intelligent and more interesting. She should watch the tracing come out of the machine with a trained, alert eye and she should be given the following practical instructions:

Notice carefully the pattern of these four leads:

1. *Lead 1:* If the complexes are inverted, check your arm electrodes—they are almost certainly reversed (fig. 21, page 33).
2. *Lead 3:* If the first deflection of the ventricular complex is downward (a Q wave), tell the patient to take a deep breath and hold it for a few heart beats (fig. 190, page 231). This may help to distinguish between important and unimportant Q waves.
3. *Lead V_1:* If the ventricular complex shows a tall upright (R) wave instead of the usual deep downstroke, take a lead or two further to the right (V_{3R}, V_{4R}) to try and get a QRS complex with the major deflection downward.
4. *Lead V_6:* If the ventricular complex shows a deep downstroke (S wave) instead of the usual tall upright wave, take a lead or two further to the left (V_7, V_8) to try and get a pattern with the major deflection upward.

Review Tracings

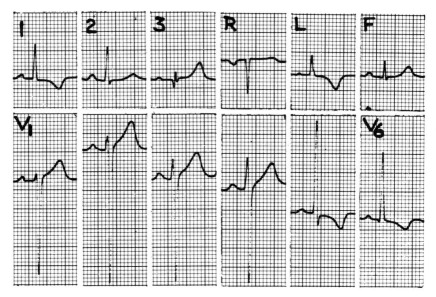

TR-1

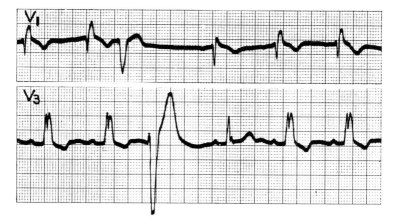

TR-2

For interpretations, see pages 314–17

Review Tracing

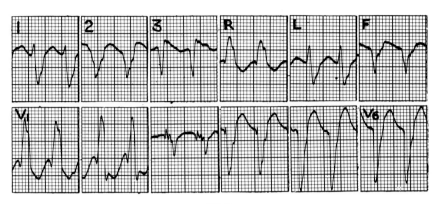

TR-3
For interpretation, see pages 314–17

11

Atrial Arrhythmias

SINUS RHYTHMS

Before dealing with the atrial arrhythmias proper, a few words should be said about the sinus (S-A) rhythms. In all of these there is normal impulse formation at the S-A node and normal spread of the impulse from there to the A-V node. The hallmark of all sinus rhythms is therefore a normal P wave.

The normal rate of impulse formation by the sinus node is generally accepted as 60 to 100 per minute. Above 100 the rhythm is called **sinus tachycardia** (fig. 96 B); below 60, **sinus bradycardia** (fig. 96 C). Sinus tachycardia results from exercise, eating, emotion, pain, hemorrhage, shock, fever, thyrotoxicosis and infections; it is a common reaction to heart disease and heart failure per se, and may be caused by many drugs, such as caffeine, nicotine, adrenaline, atropine, amyl nitrite and quinidine. Sinus bradycardia is seen as a normal variation, especially in well-trained athletes, whose heart rates may be in the thirties at rest—and often not much more with exertion; it is a physiological reaction to sleep, fright, carotid sinus massage or ocular pressure, and it may also result from disease processes, such as obstructive jaundice (effect of bile salts on sinus node), glaucoma (oculocardiac reflex), carotid sinus sensitivity and increased intracranial pressure; it is often seen in convalescence and as a result of digitalis therapy.

When the sinus node forms impulses irregularly, we have **sinus arrhythmia** (fig. 96 A). This is of two varieties: one that waxes and wanes with the phases of respiration, the heart accelerating with inspiration and slowing with expiration; and a less common type in which the changes of rate bear no relationship to the phases of respiration. Sinus arrhythmia is

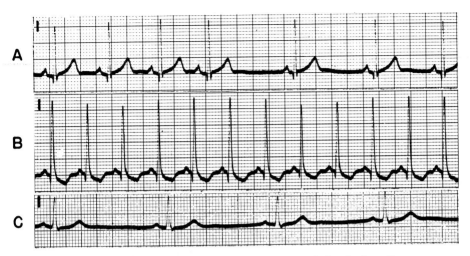

FIG. 96. A: **sinus arrhythmia.** B: **sinus tachycardia.** C: **sinus bradycardia.**

a perfectly normal finding, but it may on occasion produce such marked irregularity that it can be confused clinically with other more important arrhythmias.

THE SUPRAVENTRICULAR ARRHYTHMIAS

These arrhythmias arise from either 1) an irritable ectopic focus in the atrium, or 2) the A-V junction. They are all characterized by abnormal P waves and (unless they are complicated by coincident intraventricular block) by normal QRS duration.

ATRIAL ARRHYTHMIAS

Four atrial arrhythmias are generally described: ectopic beats, paroxysmal tachycardia, flutter and fibrillation. For some time it was thought that ectopic beats and tachycardia had a common mechanism—discharge from an irritable ectopic focus in the atrium—but that flutter and fibrillation arose by a different mechanism, namely circus movement. Prinzmetal et al. (11) presented evidence for the *"unitary nature"* of the atrial arrhythmias, demonstrating that all four arrhythmias can and probably do arise from an ectopic focus, and that circus movement is almost certainly *not* the usual underlying mechanism of any of these arrhythmias.

According to Prinzmetal's thesis, all four atrial arrhythmias have the same underlying mechanism—more or less frequent discharge of impulses from an ectopic focus in one of the atria. It appears that the most important factor in determining which arrhythmia develops is the *rate* of dis-charge from this focus. If the rate of discharge is very rapid, fibrillation results; if the rate of discharge is 300 or so, flutter is produced. If the rate is in the neighborhood of 200, paroxysmal tachycardia occurs. With rates of 100 or less, more or less frequent premature beats arise.

This simple concept has much to recommend it, besides the impressive factual evidence accumulated in its support. It leaves a few minor points unexplained, but it is overwhelmingly better and more thoroughly docu-mented than the theory of circus movement, which held almost undisputed sway for a quarter of a century.

If we accept this unitary concept, there is no fundamental difference between tachycardia and flutter; this point will be further discussed on pages 135–140.

ATRIAL PREMATURE BEATS

When an ectopic focus (i.e., a point in the atria other than the S-A node) initiates an impulse, this impulse obviously travels across the atria by an unusual path and therefore creates a distorted, often inverted, P wave. When this impulse arrives at the A-V node it will proceed down the orthodox A-V conducting paths, like any other supraventricular impulse, and, if the ventricle is not refractory, spread through and normally activate the ventricular myocardium.

We therefore recognize an ectopic atrial beat by the premature, ab-normal P wave. Such P waves are conveniently labelled P′ (P prime). Emphasis has been laid on *inversion* of the P wave. Often the ectopic P wave is inverted where it should be upright (leads 1, 2 and aVF) and up-right where it should be inverted (aVR); but this is not necessarily so and the important feature of the ectopic P is simply that its form *differs* from that of the normal P in the lead in question.

Usually the ventricles respond to the premature atrial impulse and a normal QRS-T sequence is inscribed (figs. 97 A and C, 98 A and B). If, however, the atrial impulse is very premature, so that it finds the ventric-ular conducting system still refractory, the ectopic P wave will not be fol-lowed by a ventricular complex—a "non-conducted" atrial premature beat (figs. 97 B and 98 C). In fact this is the commonest cause of a pause inter-rupting otherwise regular sinus rhythm. It is not uncommon for atrial bi-geminy to be non-conducted and so simulate an abrupt slowing of the sinus rhythm (fig. 100) until telltale P′ waves deforming the T waves (or cannon waves in the jugular pulse) indicate the true situation.

At times the impulse may find only a part of the conduction system re-fractory and so have to travel through them by an aberrant path; this re-sults in an abnormal QRS-T sequence and the phenomenon is known as

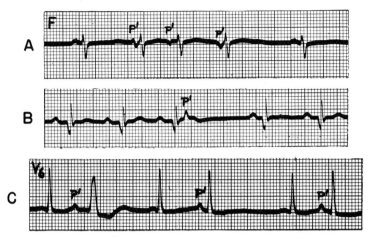

FIG. 97. **Ectopic atrial beats,** labelled P'. A. Three consecutive premature atrial beats are shown, each arising from a different atrial focus (three differently shaped P' waves). B. After the third sinus beat a very early premature beat occurs; finding the conducting tissues refractory, it is not conducted. C. **Atrial bigeminy:** every other beat is an atrial premature beat; the most premature of the three is the first, and this shows **ventricular aberration** of LBBB type.

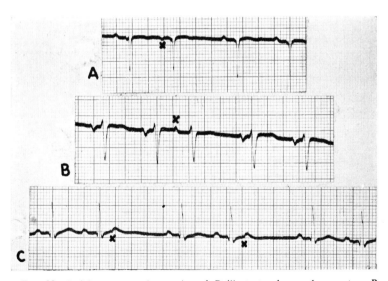

FIG. 98. **Atrial premature beats.** A and B illustrate abnormal premature P waves (x) followed by normal QRST sequences. C. Ectopic P waves are seen as notches on the T waves (x) and not followed by ventricular complexes. These are easily identifiable as abnormal P waves since the T waves of other cycles are smooth and unnotched.

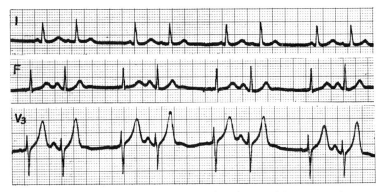

FIG. 99. **Atrial bigeminy.** Every alternate beat is an atrial premature beat producing bigeminal rhythm.

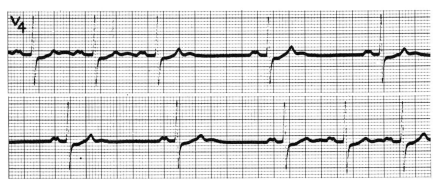

FIG. 100. Non-conducted **atrial bigeminy.** The strips are continuous. After three sinus beats, atrial bigeminy begins: the T waves of the next five beats are deformed by superimposed premature P waves whose impulses are unable to reach the ventricles.

Salient Featues of Ectopic Atrial Beats

1. Abnormal, often inverted, premature P′ wave
2. Normal QRST
3. Ensuing interval about equal to, or slightly longer than, the sinus cycle

---

** THE COMMONEST CAUSES OF PAUSES ARE NONCONDUCTED ATRIAL PREMATURE BEATS **

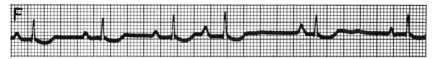

Fɪɢ. 101. **Atrial premature beat.** The 4th beat is an APB, conducted with a prolonged P-R interval. It suppresses the sinus node with the result that the postextrasystolic cycle is fully compensatory; moreover, the atrial pacemaker is shifted for the last two cycles (atrial escape beats).

aberrant ventricular conduction (6) or **ventricular aberration** (fig. 97 C). This is an important and relatively neglected subject, which is dealt with in detail in chapter 13.

The interval following an atrial premature beat is usually somewhat longer than the prevailing sinus cycle, but is usually not so long as to be *fully* compensatory (page 102). The difference in the time relationships between atrial and ventricular premature beats was illustrated in figure 70. However, ectopic impulses have a way of suppressing the sinus node (10), and if this suppressant influence is great enough, the cycle following the atrial premature beat may be fully compensatory (fig. 101) or even longer.

The atrial premature beat could, therefore, perfectly mimic the ventricular premature beat if 1) it suppressed the sinus node enough to produce a fully compensatory pause; 2) it were aberrantly conducted; and 3) the preceding P′ wave were invisible. Fortunately all three of these deviations from the norm seldom occur at once and therefore, provided the observer is on his intellectual toes, it is unlikely that an atrial premature beat can successfully masquerade as a ventricular.

ATRIAL PAROXYSMAL TACHYCARDIA

This arrhythmia can be thought of as a run of rapidly repeated premature beats. It is therefore characterized by normal QRS complexes appearing at a rapid rate, usually between 160 and 250 per minute. Their spacing is usually perfectly regular, though irregularity sometimes occurs. Theoretically an abnormal P wave precedes each QRS complex (fig. 102), but in practice the rate is usually so rapid that the P wave is merged with the preceding T wave and is indiscernible. It is therefore often impossible to distinguish between atrial and A-V nodal tachycardia and it is frequently wisest to commit oneself to the diagnosis "supraventricular tachycardia." Moreover, many "supraventricular" tachycardias are thought to be due to a circulating wave within the A-V junction (4, 14) which gives off

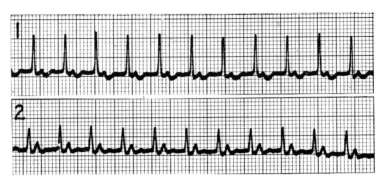

Fig. 102. **Atrial tachycardia.** Rate 170; upright P waves are clearly discernible immediately following each QRS with P-R intervals of 0.26 sec.

"daughter" waves to atria and ventricles from appropriate points in the circuit. Such a circulating wave can be initiated by an impulse originating in atria, A-V junction or ventricles. For a general discussion of this differentiation see pages 158–159.

Secondary changes in the ST-T segment may occur. Any tachycardia shortens diastole and therefore curtails coronary blood flow; if the coronaries are already diseased, and sometimes even if they are normal, ST-T changes characteristic of myocardial ischemia may develop. These changes consist of depression of the ST segment with inversion of the T wave and are well shown in figures 103 and 104. ST- and T-wave changes of this sort may persist for hours or days after the paroxysm of tachycardia has ceased, the so-called **post-tachycardia syndrome** (fig. 104).

The term **chaotic** or **multifocal atrial tachycardia** is applied when the P waves are constantly changing and the atrial rate is correspondingly irregular (7, 12). Its most common association appears to be severe pulmonary disease.

Atrial arrhythmias may be complicated by intraventricular block (fig. 105). In such circumstances the QRS complexes will obviously be prolonged, and this combination may be difficult or impossible to differentiate from ventricular tachycardia.

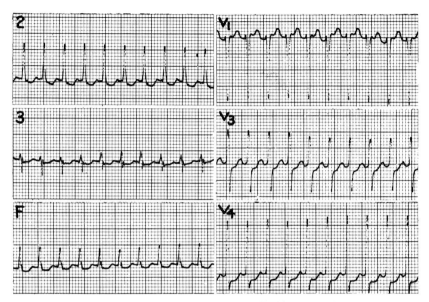

Fig. 103. **Atrial tachycardia.** Rate 230. Note normal QRS interval and ST depressions

---

Salient Features of Atrial Paroxysmal Tachycardia

1. Rapid (150–250), regular, normal QRS complexes
2. Abnormal P waves preceding QRS (rarely discernible)
3. ST-T depressions frequently seen

ATRIAL FLUTTER

Flutter versus tachycardia

According to Prinzmetal's evidence, the main difference between atrial tachycardia and flutter is that flutter represents a faster discharge from

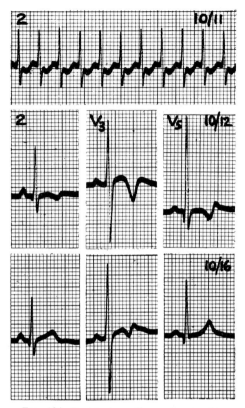

Fig. 104. **Post-tachycardia syndrome.** A paroxysm of supraventricular tachycardia is in progress in the upper strip; note associated ST depression. On the following day marked abnormalities of ST-T segments are present; these have disappeared 4 days later. From a 12-year-old boy with a normal heart.

the ectopic focus in the atrium. In the past, flutter has been arbitrarily separated from tachycardia on the basis of 1) atrial rate, 2) presence or absence of A-V block or 3) the shape of the atrial complexes.

1. An *atrial rate* of 250 has been set as the dividing line between

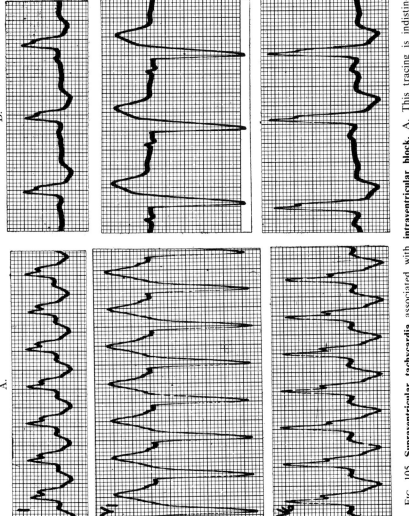

FIG. 105. **Supraventricular tachycardia** associated with **intraventricular block.** A. This tracing is indistinguishable from ventricular tachycardia. B. When sinus rhythm is later restored the QRST pattern remains virtually unchanged, proving that a supraventricular rhythm was present in A.

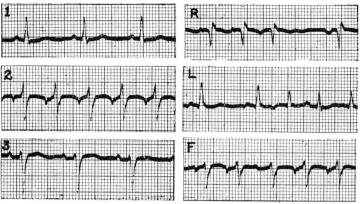

FIG. 106. **Paroxysmal atrial tachycardia.** Tracing shows onsets and endings of short bursts of atrial tachycardia. Leads 1 and 3 show normal sinus rhythm; lead 2 shows atrial tachycardia, rate 144; lead aVF also shows the tachycardia, but the third beat arises from a separate focus; lead aVR shows the last three beats of a paroxysm followed by a sinus beat; lead aVL shows two sinus beats followed by the first three beats of a paroxysm of tachycardia.

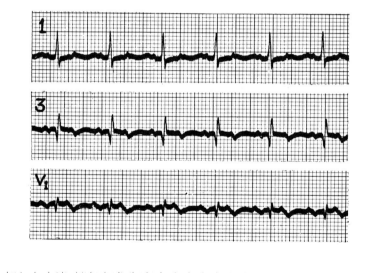

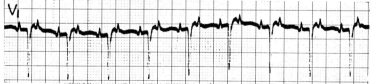

FIG. 107. Two examples of **atrial tachycardia** with 2:1 A-V block.

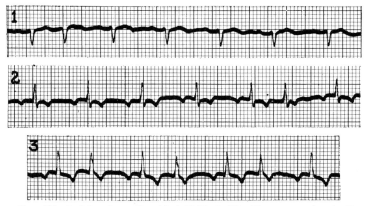

FIG. 108. **Atrial tachycardia** with A-V block. The P′ waves are barely discernible in lead 1 and are inverted in 2 and 3. The A-V block varies between 2: 1 and 3:2. In lead 3 the 3:2 ratio is constant, leaving the ventricular beats grouped in pairs—a common cause of bigeminy (see chapter 12).

tachycardia and flutter. A distinction as discretionary as a numerical boundary cannot be defended; single bouts of tachycardia have been observed in which the atrial rate has wandered on both sides of this boundary within a single uninterrupted attack.

2. The *presence of A-V block* is used by some as a criterion of flutter (see fig. 107). But it is clear that the rate at which the ventricles fail to keep pace with accelerated atria is determined by the efficiency of the A-V conducting tissues and not by the atrial mechanism. Block will not develop in one heart till a rate of, say, 250 is attained, whereas it may develop at 200 in another. By the criterion of block the rhythm will still be called paroxysmal tachycardia at 240 in the first heart, while at 210 in the second heart it will already be flutter—simply because the second heart has a less efficient A-V conducting system.

3. The *form of the P waves* is perhaps the most characteristic of the traditional criteria for diagnosing flutter. As far as we know at present, the shape and direction of abnormal atrial waves depend mainly on two factors: the *part* of the atrium in which the ectopic focus is situated, and the *rate* of discharge from that focus. Apparently, the faster the rate of discharge, the more likely is the atrial wave to become distorted into the form that we have come to regard as typical of flutter. This is not the whole story, however, for the typical contour of flutter waves may be seen at times at an atrial rate of no more than 200, whereas the small abnormal complexes usually associated with paroxysmal tachycardia may be seen at rates near 300. Furthermore, these complexes may have

the one form in one lead and the other in another lead in the same tracing.

In view of these considerations it is arbitrary and illogical to separate
flutter from tachycardia on the basis of rate, presence of A-V block or
form of the atrial complexes. Opponents of the "unitary" concept, however, further point out that flutter is more common in elderly patients
with heart disease, whereas tachycardia is more common in the young
and healthy; that tachycardia more often begins in the cephalic region
of the atria whereas flutter more often originates caudally; and that,
whereas vagal stimulation frequently abolishes tachycardia, it usually
has little effect on flutter and many indeed convert it to fibrillation. These
arguments are of importance but, as tachycardia and flutter cannot be
clearly and exclusively defined, distinctions such as these cannot with certainty be attributed to either of them. It is therefore more logical to lump
them together as paroxysmal tachycardia, with or without A-V block.
As this revision of nomenclature has not yet been widely accepted, for
the present it seems wisest to include in this section a description of the
traditional pattern of flutter.

Classical flutter

Typical atrial flutter (figs. 109–115) is recognized by the presence of
"saw-tooth" or undulating atrial waves, with ventricular responses following every 2nd, 3rd, 4th, (up to 8th) atrial wave. These waves have
been labelled "F" (for flutter) waves. These waves do not reveal themselves with equal clarity in all leads: leads 2 and 3 usually show flutter
waves most clearly, while lead 1 may be particularly treacherous in giving virtually no evidence of the typical pattern (fig. 114). The most common rate of flutter waves is between 300 and 320 with 2:1 conduction producing therefore a ventricular rate of 150 to 160 (figs. 109 and 110).

The QRS complex, as with all atrial arrhythmias, is of normal duration unless intraventricular block coincidentally complicates the picture.
The T wave is usually dominated by the zigzagging atrial complexes so
that it is not clearly identifiable, but it often distorts the otherwise
uniform saw-tooth pattern.

Analysis of flutter waves

The saw-tooth waves of flutter have been interestingly analyzed by
Prinzmetal. He has demonstrated that the downward deflection is the
abnormal P (P') wave and is followed by an upward Ta (or T$_P$) wave,

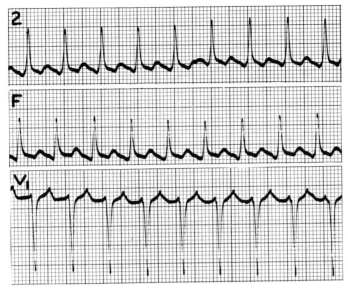

Fig. 109. **Atrial flutter** with 2:1 A-V conduction—the commonest ratio.

Salient Features of Atrial Flutter

1. "Saw-tooth" or undulating baseline of "F" waves
2. Normal QRS complexes in 2:1 to 8:1 ratio
3. T waves swamped by the F wave pattern

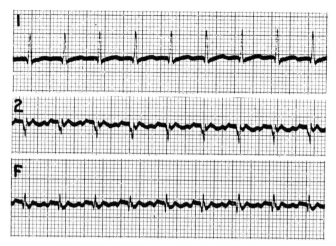

FIG. 110. **Atrial flutter** with 2:1 A-V conduction

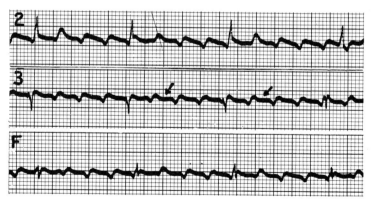

FIG. 111. **Atrial flutter** with 4:1 A-V conduction—the second most common ratio. Note the "saw-tooth" effect and the isoelectric "shelf" (arrows) between F waves.

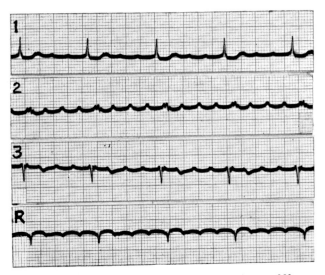

FIG. 112. **Atrial flutter** with 4:1 A-V block. Atrial rate 252, ventricular rate 63. This patient would present clinically with an unsuspicious regular rhythm with heart rate in the sixties; but the diagnosis might be made if the neck veins were carefully inspected for the rapid flutter waves.

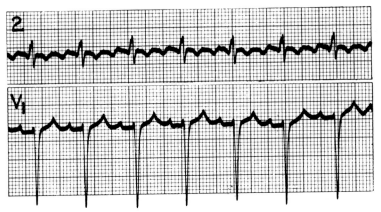

FIG. 113. **Atrial flutter** with 3:1 A-V block—a rare ratio

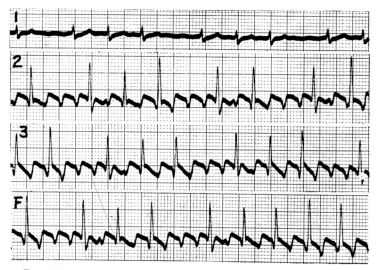

FIG. 114. **Atrial flutter** with A-V conduction varying between 2:1 and 4:1. Notice lack of evidence of atrial activity in lead 1.

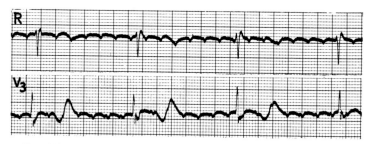

FIG. 115. **Atrial flutter** with complete A-V block. The atrial rate is about 280 and the F waves change their relationship to the QRS complexes, which are independently regular at a rate of 45. Note the monstrous T-U complex in V_3.

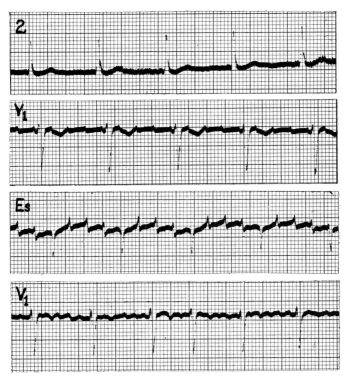

F<small>IG</small>. 116. **Atrial flutter** with 4:1 A-V block. The only routine lead that showed any sign of atrial activity was V_1. The third strip (Es) is an esophageal lead. The fourth strip is V_1 after digitalization, showing **atrial fibrillation.**

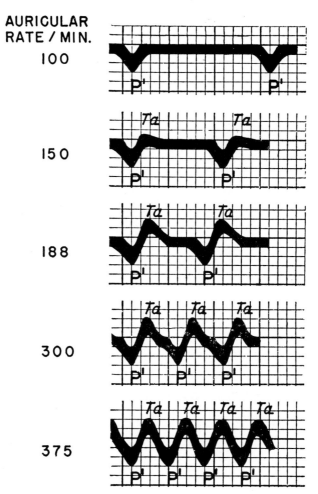

FIG. 117. Illustrating that with increase in rate 1) the Ta wave assumes greater prominence and 2) the isoelectric shelf becomes shorter. Reproduced with kind permission of the publishers from *The Auricular Arrhythmias*, by Myron Prinzmetal and others, Charles C Thomas, 1951).

i.e., the wave of atrial repolarization. This rapid P′-Ta sequence is followed by a horizontal isoelectric pause before the next P′ wave begins. The length of this pause is determined by atrial rate, becoming longer as the rate slows, and disappearing altogether at very rapid rates. He has termed this interval the **isoelectric shelf,** and it is shown in figure 111. Figure 117 illustrates diagrammatically both the development of Ta waves and the shortening of the isoelectric shelf as the rate increases.

ATRIAL FIBRILLATION

When the ectopic discharge becomes excessively rapid, it also becomes irregular. It no longer leaves a regular imprint on the electrocardiogram and it no longer elicits a regular ventricular response. The uneven and irregular deviations in the tracing that now represent atrial activity are labelled "f" waves (figs. 118–120). At times no sign at all of atrial activity is visible in the routine leads, and then the diagnosis can be inferred from the irregular ventricular response in the apparent absence of atrial activity.

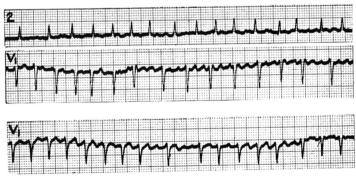

FIG. 118. **Atrial fibrillation.** Two examples with rapid irregular ventricular response.

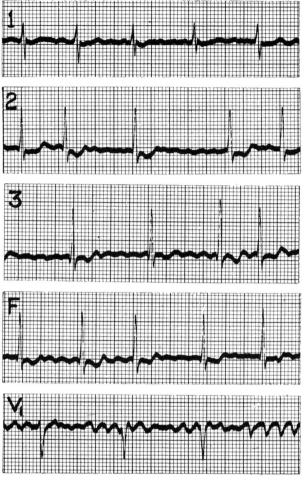

FIG. 119. **Atrial fibrillation.** The typical, uneven, irregular
"f" waves are visible in all leads.

Salient Features of Atrial Fibrillation

1. Absence of P waves, which are replaced by irregular "f" waves (or no sign at all of atrial activity)
2. Normal QRS complexes, irregular in time and
   sometimes varying in amplitude

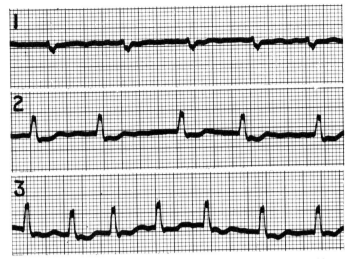

FIG. 120. **Atrial fibrillation** with right axis deviation; this combination is highly suspicious of mitral stenosis.

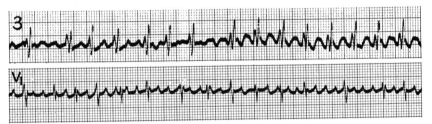

FIG. 121. Two examples of **atrial flutter-fibrillation.** The atrial waves are too well formed and regular to be called unqualified fibrillation, yet not regular enough to be pure flutter.

Sometimes a mixture of fibrillation with flutter is seen, as in figure 121, and may be called **flutter-fibrillation** or **impure flutter.**

Just as the ventricles have a vulnerable period, so there is a point in the atrial cycle at which an atrial premature impulse is likely to precipitate an atrial tachyarrhythmia. Killip has formularized the situation as follows: if the P-P′ interval (i.e., the interval from the preceding P wave to the pre-

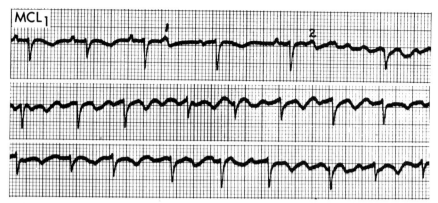

FIG. 122. **Atrial fibrillation** precipitated by APB (2) in top strip. The first APB (1) ends a cycle more than half the preceding cycle; whereas the second APB (2) ends a cycle less than half the preceding P-P interval, therefore lands in the "vulnerable phase" of the atrial cycle and precipitates fibrillation.

mature P' wave) is less than half the preceding P-P interval, it is likely to land in the vulnerable period and spark a tachyarrhythmia; but if the P-P' interval is more than 60 per cent of the preceding P-P interval, it is unlikely to do so (6) (fig. 122).

The irregularity of fibrillation may be clinically imitated by five other arrhythmias:

1. Frequent ectopic beats—ventricular, atrial or A-V nodal. These often produce a pulse deficit. Note that a pulse deficit is *not* diagnostic of atrial fibrillation.
2. Atrial tachycardia (flutter) with varying A-V block.
3. Sinus rhythm with varying A-V block.
4. Gross sinus arrhythmia.
5. Wandering pacemaker.

The important causes of atrial fibrillation are rheumatic heart disease with mitral valve involvement, coronary disease, hypertension and thyrotoxicosis; it not uncommonly complicates constrictive pericarditis and atrial septal defect. At times it is found in apparently healthy hearts (3).

REFERENCES

1. Dressler, W.: Prolonged depressing effect of premature supraventricular beats. Am. Heart J. 1966: **72**, 25.
2. Enselberg, C. D.: The esophageal electrocardiogram in the study of atrial activity and cardiac arrhythmias. Am. Heart J. 1951: **41**, 382.
3. Evans, W., and Swann, P.: Lone auricular fibrillation. Brit. Heart J. 1954: **16**, 189.

4. Gettes, A., et al.: Depression of cardiac pacemakers by premature impulses. Am. Heart J. 1951: **41**, 49.

5. Killip, T., and Gault, J. H.: Mode of onset of atrial fibrillation in man. Am. Heart J. 1965: **70**, 172.

6. Langendorf, R.: Aberrant ventricular conduction. Am. Heart J. 1951: **41**, 700.

7. Lipson, M. J., and Naimi, S.: Multifocal atrial tachycardia (chaotic atrial tachycardia). Clinical associations and significance. Circulation 1970: **42**, 397.

8. Lown, B., et al.: Interrelationship of digitalis and potassium in auricular tachycardia with block. Am. Heart J. 1953: **45**, 589.

9. Lown, B., et al.: Paroxysmal atrial tachycardia with block. Circulation 1960: **21**, 129.

10. Pick, A., et al.: Depression of cardiac pacemakers by premature impulses. Am. Heart J. 1951: **41**, 49.

11. Prinzmetal, M., et al.: *The Auricular Arrhythmias.* Charles C Thomas, Springfield, Ill., 1952.

12. Shine, K. I., et al.: Multifocal atrial tachycardia. Clinical and electrocardiographic features in 32 patients. New Eng. J. Med. 1968: **279**, 344.

13. Simonson, E., and Berman, R.: Differentiation between paroxysmal auricular tachycardia with partial A-V block and auricular flutter. Am. Heart J. 1951: **42**, 387.

14. Wellens, H. J. J.: *Electrical Stimulation of the Heart in the Study and Treatment of Tachycardias.* University Park Press, Baltimore, 1971.

Review Tracings

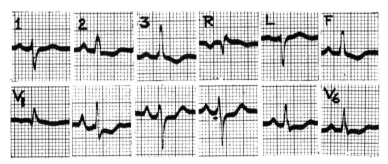

TR-4

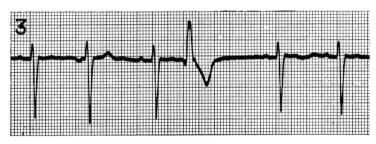

TR-5

For interpretations, see pages 314–17

Review Tracing

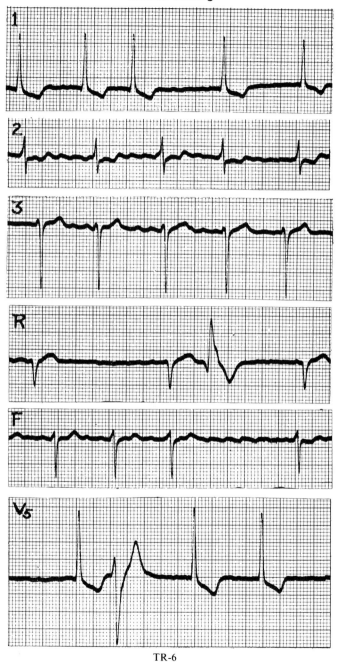

TR-6
For interpretation, see pages 314–17

12

A-V Nodal (Junctional) Arrhythmias

Investigating physiologists have been unable to demonstrate pacemaking cells in the A-V node proper, though they found them in the His bundle and the junction between node and bundle (3). For this reason the propriety of the terms "A-V nodal" and "nodal" to describe arrhythmias is open to question, and some authorities are at pains to avoid nodal and to use "A-V" or "junctional." Since the matter is still sub judice and "nodal" is well entrenched, shorter and more euphonious than "junctional", I have not abandoned "nodal" and shall continue to use interchangeably "A-V nodal," "nodal," "A-V junctional," "junctional," and also simply "A-V," which is noncommittal and has enjoyed the blessing of uninterrupted usage since 1915.

A-V PREMATURE BEATS AND TACHYCARDIA—
A-V RHYTHM

When the impulse arises in the A-V junction, it travels up through the atria and down through the ventricles more or less simultaneously. The impulse travels down to the ventricles by its normal paths, and therefore the QRST sequence is normal; but it is travelling in reverse through the atria and therefore the P wave is distorted ("retrograde P wave"), being inverted in several leads where it should be upright. The axis of the P wave is in the neighborhood of −90°; i.e., it is nearly isoelectric in 1, frankly inverted in 2, 3 and aVF, and upright in aVR and aVL. Three varieties of this pattern may occur:

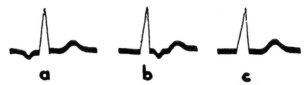

FIG. 123. A-V nodal patterns. a. Abnormal "retrograde" P wave precedes QRS with short P-R interval (upper nodal rhythm). b. Abnormal P wave follows QRS (lower nodal rhythm). c. P wave coincides with QRS and is lost (mid-nodal rhythm).

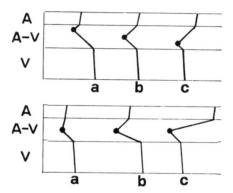

FIG. 124. In the upper diagram the concept of "upper," and "mid-" and "lower" **nodal rhythm** is depicted. The impulse travels at a uniform rate in each direction so that if it begins high in the node (a) the atria will be activated before the ventricles; if it begins midway down the node (b) both will be activated simultaneously; and if it begins low down (c) the ventricles will be activated before the atria. In the bottom diagram the impulse is portrayed as arising at the same level in the node, but its rate of travel varies: with normal rapid spread in both directions (a) the atria are activated slightly before the ventricles; with equally delayed conduction in both directions (b) the atria will still be activated first; if forward conduction is normal but retrograde conduction is delayed (c) the ventricles will be activated before the atria and the P' wave will be inscribed *after* the QRS.

1. If the impulse reaches and spreads through the atria first, the abnormal P wave closely precedes the QRS complex (fig. 123a), the P-R interval being shorter than normal.
2. If the impulse reaches the ventricles first, the abnormal P wave is inscribed following the QRS (fig. 123b).
3. If the impulse spreads through atria and ventricles simultaneously, the P wave is lost in the QRS (fig. 123c).

For descriptive purposes these three varieties are known respectively as upper (or high), lower (or low), and mid-nodal rhythm; although, in fact, it is probably not the level in the node at which the impulse arises that deter-

Salient Features of A-V Nodal Rhythms

1. Abnormal P waves closely preceding or following QRS; or absent P waves
2. Normal QRST sequence

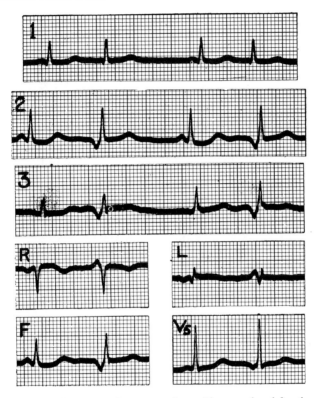

FIG. 125. **A-V nodal premature beats.** The second and fourth beats in leads 1, 2 and 3 are high nodal premature beats, producing nodal bigeminy. In the remaining leads the second beat is a nodal beat. Note the short P-R interval in the nodal beat (0.09 sec.). The retrograde P waves are inverted in 2, 3, aVF and V_5, upright in aVR and aVL and isoelectric in 1.

mines whether the atria or ventricles are first activated, but rather the rate of spread in both directions, presence of block, and so on. The two concepts are contrasted diagrammatically in figure 124. The A-V node may initiate a single such beat, an **A-V nodal premature beat** (figs. 125–127).

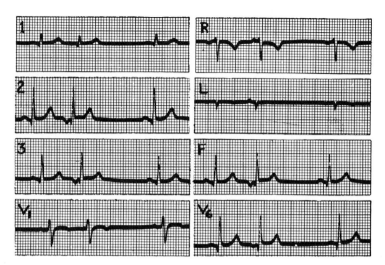

FIG. 126. **A-V nodal premature beats.** Each lead contains a high nodal premature beat between two normal sinus beats. P-R interval of nodal beats is about 0.10 sec.

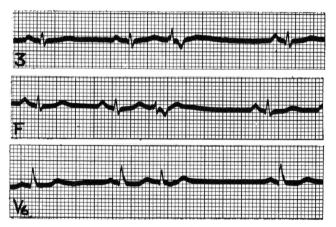

FIG. 127. **A-V nodal premature beats.** The third beat in each lead is a low nodal premature beat—the P wave *follows* the QRS. The QRS complexes of the premature beats show some degree of ventricular aberration.

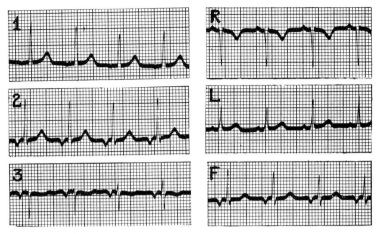

FIG. 128. **A-V nodal tachycardia,** rate about 102. Note short P-R interval with inverted P waves in 2, 3 and aVF with upright P waves in aVR.

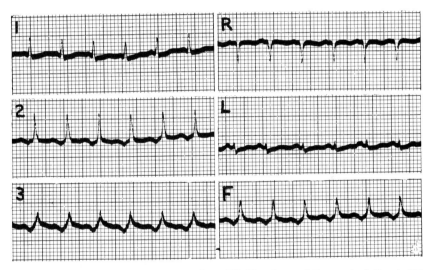

FIG. 129. **A-V nodal tachycardia,** rate about 170. Note inverted P waves in 2, 3 and aVF, upright in aVR; the P-R interval is 0.09 sec.

Sometimes the A-V pacemaker becomes exceedingly irritable and initiates a paroxysm of tachycardia, **A-V nodal tachycardia** (figs. 128–131). When the S-A node is suppressed by drugs or disease, or is congenitally absent, the A-V node may come to the rescue and act as the pacemaker of the

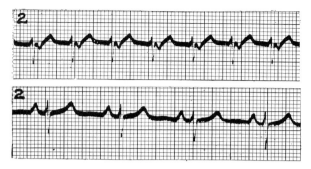

FIG. 130. **A-V nodal tachycardia.** Two strips of lead 2 taken 10 min. apart: upper strip shows nodal tachycardia with retrograde P waves; lower strip shows normal sinus rhythm restored after 20 mg. methoxamine intravenously.

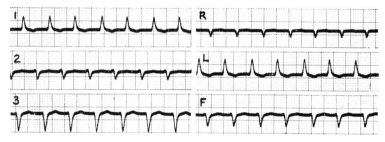

FIG. 131. **A-V nodal tachycardia,** rate about 144. P waves are not seen and are presumably lost within the QRS complexes; this is therefore compatible with a "mid-nodal" tachycardia; but it could just as well be a sinus or atrial tachycardia with long P-R interval and with the P wave buried in the preceding QRS complex.

heart in its own intrinsic rhythm (35 to 60 beats per minute)—**A-V nodal rhythm** (fig. 132). All of these rhythms are relatively uncommon.

The A-V nodal premature beat with the preceding P wave can be distinguished from an atrial premature beat only by the shortened P-R interval. Similarly A-V nodal tachycardia can be distinguished from atrial tachycardia only if the abnormal P wave is clearly visible and accompanied by a shortened P-R interval; otherwise the distinction is often difficult or impossible. If the P-wave pattern is typically nodal and associated with a normal or prolonged P-R interval, one cannot be sure whether the rhythm is ectopic atrial (perhaps coronary sinus; see below) or A-V nodal with some degree of forward A-V block. Again, if typical P waves closely *follow* the QRS (as in fig. 130), unless one is lucky enough to record the first or last beat of the paroxysm, one can never be sure whether the rhythm is "lower" nodal or whether the ectopic atrial impulse is conducted to the *next* QRS with prolonged A-V conduction—for such prolongation is common

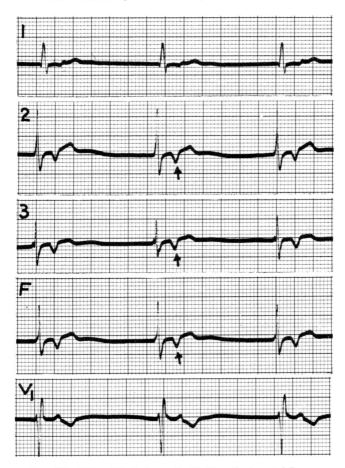

Fig. 132. **A-V nodal rhythm,** rate 47. Note the inverted P waves (arrows) following the QRS in 2, 3 and aVF with upright P waves in V₁.

at rapid rates. In this dilemma, it is more honest to settle for a diagnosis of "supraventricular" tachycardia.

CORONARY NODAL RHYTHM

When the P waves and QRS complexes are normal but the P-R interval is abnormally short (less than 0.12 sec.), some authorities have applied the term **coronary nodal rhythm** (3, 6). Others call it the Lown-Ganong-Levine (or L-G-L) syndrome (7). Its mechanism and full significance are not clear, but its owners sometimes have hypertension and a predisposition to atrial tachycardia.

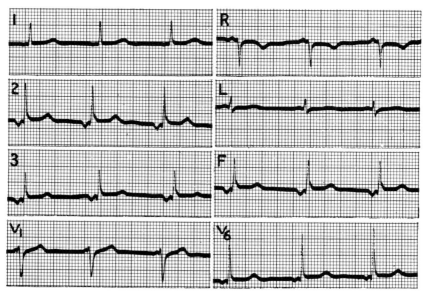

Fig. 133. **A-V nodal rhythm,** rate 66. Note inverted P waves preceding QRS in 2, 3, aVF and V$_6$, with upright P waves in aVR and V$_1$. P-R interval is 0.10 sec.

CORONARY SINUS RHYTHMS

When P waves have the same shape and direction as those of A-V nodal rhythm but are associated with a normal (rather than short) P-R interval, there is reason to believe that such beats are likely to arise from the neighborhood of the coronary sinus. Scherf et al. (11, 12) have applied the terms **coronary sinus rhythm** and **coronary sinus extrasystoles** to arrhythmias showing these features (fig. 134). There is little doubt, however, that such a combination can also indicate a *left atrial* origin.

LEFT ATRIAL RHYTHMS

Another development has upset our time-honored concepts of A-V nodal rhythm. Mirowski has drawn attention to the fact that we have based our diagnosis of A-V nodal activity on the P-wave pattern in the limb leads alone and ignored their morphology in the chest leads. He maintains that many of the rhythms that we call "nodal" are really of left atrial origin and he suggests that an important criterion for left atrial rhythm is an in-

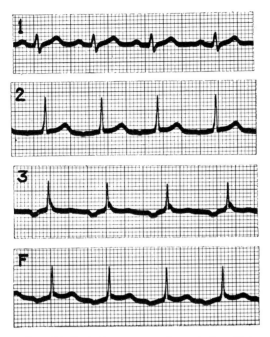

FIG. 134. Probable **coronary sinus rhythm.** Note inverted P waves in 2, 3 and aVF with P-R interval at upper limit of normal (0.20 sec.).

verted P wave in V_6 as in figure 133, often associated with an upright P wave in V_1 (10). His argument does not explain why "left atrial" rhythms should so often have short P-R intervals, and for the moment the matter must remain unsettled. Meanwhile he has done us a service in focussing attention on the precordial P waves in tracings that show typical "retrograde" P waves in the limb leads.

According to others, the most persuasive index of left atrial rhythm is an inverted P wave in lead 1 (1, 14).

WANDERING PACEMAKER

Rarely the site of impulse formation may vary between S-A and A-V nodes, some beats arising from one and some from the other, often with intervening atrial fusion beats. This phenomenon is known as **wandering** or

shifting pacemaker (figs. 135, 136). A shift in pacemaker is often precipitated by a premature beat (fig. 137). The term is *not* applied to the change in pacemaker activity inherent in atrial or A-V premature beats.

MAIN-STEM EXTRASYSTOLES

When a premature beat of supraventricular form is associated with no disturbance in shape or rhythm of P waves and is followed by a fully compensatory pause, it was assumed that the beat arose in the main stem of

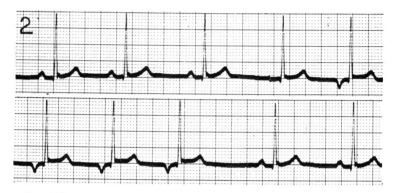

FIG. 135. **Wandering** or **shifting pacemaker.** The two strips are continuous. The first three beats are sinus beats; then comes an atrial fusion beat followed by four A-V nodal beats, and then the pacemaker shifts back to the S-A node for the last two beats.

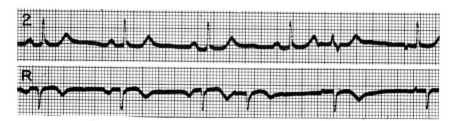

FIG. 136. A **shift of pacemaker** induced by an APB in each lead.

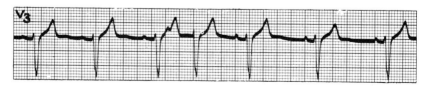

FIG. 137. The fourth beat is an atrial extrasystole—the P′ wave deforms the upstroke of the T wave and is conducted with a prolonged P-R interval. Following the premature beat, the P waves change and the rate slows, indicating a shift of pacemaker.

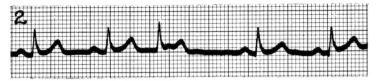

FIG. 138. **A-V junctional premature beat** without retrograde conduction to the atria. The third beat is premature and has a normal shape. A rhythmic sinus P wave is seen deforming the ST segment of the premature beat. The pause following the premature beat is fully compensatory.

the bundle of His and it was called a mainstem extrasystole (8) (fig. 138). Such a beat thus has features of both ventricular and supraventricular premature beats—in form it is like a supraventricular beat, but the undisturbed sequence of P waves and the compensatory pause are points in common with ventricular beats.

The assumption that such beats arose in the main stem was tenuous. However, in view of the physiological studies referred to above, it may well be that most or all of the beats we call A-V nodal actually arise in the His bundle.

HIS BUNDLE RECORDINGS

His bundle electrography in man (2) is an exciting development for those with a special interest in arrhythmias and conduction disturbances. By proper positioning of a multipolar electrode catheter, it is possible to obtain simultaneous recordings of the electrical activity of the A-V node, the bundle of His and the right bundle branch. Thus for the first time we are able to some extent to dissect and partition the P-R interval into two stages: from atrium to bundle of His (A-H interval); and from bundle of His to ventricles (H-V interval). This has proved instructive in elucidating the mechanisms of A-V block.

The main contribution of the technique to date is in confirming assumptions already ingeniously deduced from clinical tracings—it has converted the game of inference into a science. It has confirmed the fact that concealed retrograde conduction follows ectopic ventricular beats; that concealed A-V junctional extrasystoles exist and can mimic first and second degree A-V block; and that patterns of concealed conduction into the A-V junction account for the irregular ventricular response to atrial fibrillation.

But in addition to its role in confirmation, it has also provided a fresh approach to arrhythmia research; and, when all else fails, it may be the only means of resolving a difficult arrhythmia. For example, a His bundle recording alone may settle the notoriously difficult differentiation between ventricular aberration and ectopy, since ventricular complexes that result from supraventricular impulses must be preceded by His bundle activation, whereas ectopic ventricular complexes are not. Again, by this technique it has been demonstrated that the site of conduction delay during Wenckebach periodicity is in the A-V node itself (prolongation of A-H interval) whereas in type II 2nd degree A-V block, the site of block is below the bundle of His (prolongation of H-V interval). Finally, the technique has yielded precise and useful information concerning the action of antiarrhythmic drugs on A-V conduction.

COMPARISON OF THE THREE MAIN TYPES OF PREMATURE BEATS

In figure 139 seven possible variations on the extrasystolic theme are graphically represented. The numbers of these seven beats are circled; the others are all sinus beats with a normal A-V sequence.

The first premature beat (**3**) is a premature ventricular beat followed by a compensatory pause (fig. 70 A, page 103). The second premature beat (**5**) is similar, but is even more premature; it is so premature that the next sinus beat finds the ventricle recovered and so initiates a normal ventricular contraction. Such a premature beat, shoved in between two normal beats with no compensatory pause, is an interpolated premature beat (fig. 72). The third premature beat (**7**) is barely premature; the impulse has already spread through the atria, and the ventricular ectopic focus only just casts its vote in time (fig. 71 B). The next premature beat (**9**) is atrial, with normal A-V sequence, and is followed·by an approximately normal cardiac cycle. The next three premature beat (**11, 12, 13**) are A-V nodal; in **12** the impulse spreads through atria and ventricles simultaneously; in **11** it traverses atria before ventricles (fig. 126, page 156), and in **13** ventricles before atria (fig. 127).

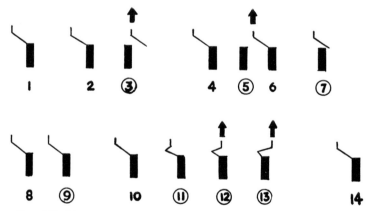

FIG. 139. Diagram of atrio-ventricular relationships in various forms of premature beats (see text). The arrows indicate cannon waves.

Ventricular contraction closes the A-V valves. Therefore, in those premature beats where the ventricles contract *simultaneously with* or *before* the atria, i.e., beats **3, 5, 12** and **13** the subsequent atrial contraction vainly throws the blood against closed A-V valves; in such circumstances there is no escape for the blood in the right atrium but back into the veins. This may often be seen in an accentuated venous "a" wave in the neck, a **cannon wave.** Thus in some ventricular (**3** and **5**) and some A-V nodal (**12** and **13**) beats cannon waves may be seen, but they are *not* seen in atrial premature beats (**9**), where normal A-V sequence is undisturbed—*unless* the atrial beat is so premature that atrial contraction occurs before the tricuspid valve has opened; then the cannon wave *precedes* the early ventricular contraction.

REFERENCES

1. Bix, H. H.: The electrocardiographic pattern of initial stimulation in the left auricle. Sinai Hosp. J. 1953: **2**, 37.
2. Damato, A. N., and Lau, S. H.: Clinical value of the electrogram of the conduction system. Prog. Cardiovasc. Dis. 1970: **13**, 119.
3. Eyring, E. J., and Spodick, D. H.: Coronary nodal rhythm. Am. J. Cardiol. 1960: **5**, 781.
4. Fisch, C., and Knoebel, S. B.: Junctional rhythms. Progr. Cardiovasc. Dis. 1970: **13**, 141.
5. Hoffman, B. F., and Cranefield, P. F.: The physiological basis of cardiac arrhythmias. Am. J. Med. 1964: **37**, 670.
6. Katz, L. N., and Pick, A.: *Clinical Electrocardiography. The Arrhythmias.* Lea and Febiger Philadelphia, 1956.
7. Lown, B., et al.: The syndrome of the short P-R interval normal QRS complex and paroxysmal rapid heart action. Circulation 1952: **5**, 693.
8. Marriott, H. J. L., and Bradley, S. M.: Main-stem extrasystoles. Circulation 1957; **16**, 544.
9. Marriott, H. J. L.: Nodal mechanisms with dependent activation of atria and ventricles. In *Mechanisms and Therapy of Cardiac Arrhythmias*, 14th Hahnemann Symposium, Grune and Stratton, New York, 1966.
10. Mirowski, M.: Left atrial rhythm. Diagnostic criteria and differentiation from nodal arrhythmias. Am. J. Cardiol. 1966: **17**, 203.
11. Scherf, D., and Gurbuzer, B.: Further studies on coronary sinus rhythm. Am. J. Cardiol. 1958: **16**, 579.
12. Scherf, D., and Harris, R.: Coronary sinus rhythm. Am. Heart J. 1946: **32**, 443.
13. Scherf, D., and Cohen, J.: *The Atrioventricular Node and Selected Cardiac Arrhythmias.* Grune and Stratton, New York, 1964.
14. Somlyo, A. P., and Grayzel, J.: Left atrial arrhythmias. Am. Heart J. 1963: **65**, 68.
15. Spodick, D. H., and Colman, R.: Observations on coronary sinus rhythm and its mechanism. Am. J. Cardiol. 1961: **7**, 198.

Review Tracings

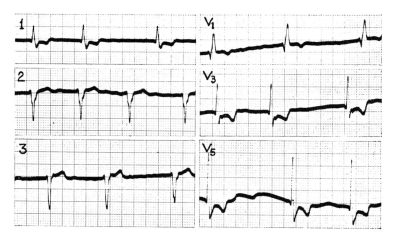

TR-7

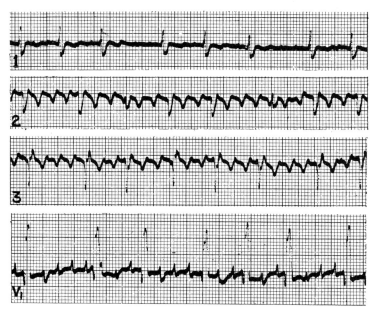

TR-8
For interpretations, see pages 314–17

Review Tracing

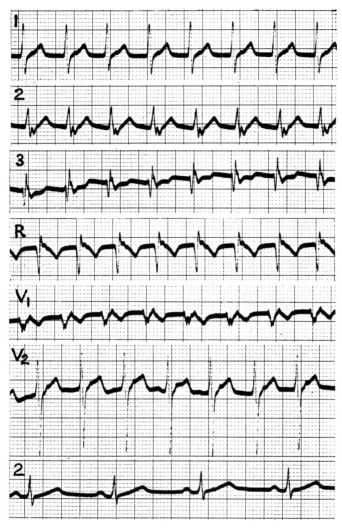

TR-9
For interpretation, see pages 314–17

13

Aberrant Ventricular Conduction
and the Diagnosis of Tachycardia

Things are seldom what they seem,
Skim milk masquerades as cream.—*Gilbert*

Aberrant ventricular conduction, or ventricular aberration, is an important subject deserving detailed treatment. Its importance rests firmly on two facts: 1) it is common—much commoner than most interpreters realize; 2) it is often overlooked with the result that supraventricular arrhythmias are frequently misdiagnosed as ventricular, and this has important therapeutic implications.

If its existence is appreciated at all, ventricular aberration is generally regarded as a relative curiosity and left for the experts in arrhythmias to worry with. This is unrealistic. Almost all physicians are occasionally called upon to diagnose and treat paroxysmal tachycardia and atrial fibrillation; and they should presumably, therefore, know something of the fundamental differentiation between supraventricular and ventricular tachycardias.

The dilemma arises in those tachycardias with widened, bizarre QRS complexes, which therefore have the appearance of ventricular tachycardia. It is generally assumed that such tachycardias are in fact ventricular "until proved otherwise." This is a conventional dogma that can lead to upwards of a 50 per cent error in the diagnosis of a certain group of tachycardias, and it is therefore unsound teaching. There is a surprisingly good chance that such an arrhythmia is indeed supraventricular and that the anomalous complexes are the result of aberrant ventricular conduction.

If a supraventricular impulse arrives so early that the A-V node or bundle, or both bundle branches, are still in their refractory period, the beat will not be conducted to the ventricles. On the other hand, if it arrives after the entire conducting system has recovered from the previous beat, the impulse will be normally conducted. If it arrives somewhere between these two extremes and finds part of the conducting system recovered but part still refractory, it will be conducted abnormally (aberrantly) through the ventricles. Most commonly it is part of the right bundle-branch system that is found refractory so that most aberrant patterns are of right bundle-branch block form.

The refractory period of the conducting paths is proportional to the length of the preceding cycle (R-R interval); i.e., the longer the cycle and slower the rate, the longer the refractory period, and vice versa. Ventricular aberration can therefore result either from shortening of the immediate cycle or by lengthening of the preceding one, or by a combination of both (fig. 140).

Figures 141–151 illustrate aberrant conduction occurring in various supraventricular arrhythmias, and the pertinent points in diagnosis are dealt with in the respective legends. From a study of these figures it should be

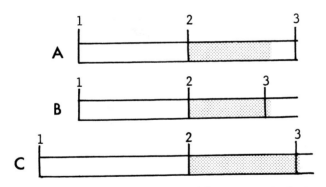

Fig. 140. In the diagrams, 1, 2 and 3 are consecutive beats and the stippled area represents the refractory period of some part of the conducting system during the second cycle. In A, there are two regular cycles with normal conduction. Beat 3 may become aberrant (lower two diagrams) if either the first cycle is lengthened or the second cycle is shortened. Shortening of the second cycle (B) may bring the beat within the refractory period of part of the conducting system; lengthening of the preceding cycle (C) will prolong the refractory period so that the next beat, though no earlier than before, falls within the now longer refractory period. (Reproduced from Marriott, *Armchair Arrhythmias*. Tampa Tracings, 1965.)

evident that confusion can readily occur and that such confusion can have serious consequences.

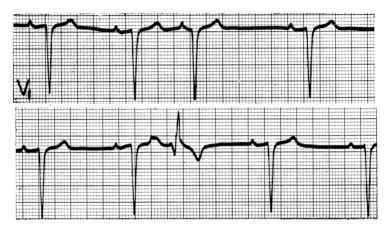

FIG. 141. **Atrial premature beats.** The third beat in each strip is an atrial premature beat; in the upper strip the ectopic P wave is clearly visible and is followed by normal conduction to the ventricles. In the lower strip the ectopic beat is much more premature (P wave deforms upstroke of T wave) and finds the right bundle branch still refractory, so that "ventricular aberration" of RBBB type occurs. This beat might easily be mistaken for an ectopic *ventricular* beat.

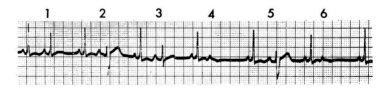

FIG. 142. **Atrial bigeminy.** Ectopic atrial beats are numbered 1 to 6. Beats 4 and 6 are so premature that they are not conducted to the ventricles. Beats 2 and 5 are not quite so premature, yet they find part of the ventricular conduction system still refractory and are conducted with ventricular aberration. Beat 3 is conducted with only minor aberration, and beat 1 shows almost normal intraventricular conduction.

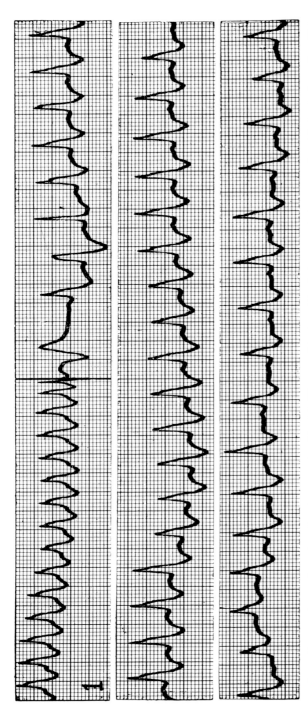

Fig. 143. **Ventricular aberration.** Continuous strip of lead 1. The record begins with what appears to be a run of ventricular tachycardia. Clinically at rate 245 the first heart sound was constant and there were no irregular cannon waves. After procaine amide the paroxysm gives place to a sinus tachycardia, in which the preceding P waves are well seen at the end of the bottom strip. Because the ventricular complexes are identical with those shown during the paroxysmal tachycardia (beginning of top strip), there can be no doubt that the paroxysm was of supraventricular origin with aberrant ventricular conduction.

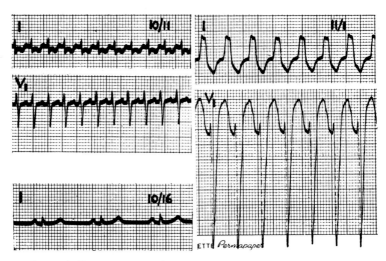

FIG. 144. Two paroxysms of **tachycardia** in a boy of 12 with no demonstrable heart disease. At left the paroxysm is unmistakably supraventricular. At the right, three weeks later, the QRS pattern has altered markedly and now appears to represent ventricular tachycardia at a considerably slower rate. However, the first heart sound was constant and a lead S_5 demonstrated P waves in relation to each QRS complex. Supraventricular tachycardia with aberrant ventricular conduction is therefore the more likely diagnosis (the only possible alternative being ventricular tachycardia with retrograde conduction to the atria).

Conclusion to legend to figure 145

tory. This is then a supraventricular premature beat with aberration, and the aberrant complex is identical with the ventricular complexes during the paroxysm in the upper lead 2 (second strip). In aVF (fifth strip) there are two couplets of atrial bigeminy followed by two triplets of atrial trigeminy. In these triplets, the second premature beat shows ventricular aberration with bizarre complexes identical with the QRS complexes during the paroxysm in the upper lead aVF (third strip). All of this adds up to overwhelming evidence that the "ventricular" tachycardia in the upper three strips is really supraventricular with aberrant ventricular conduction.

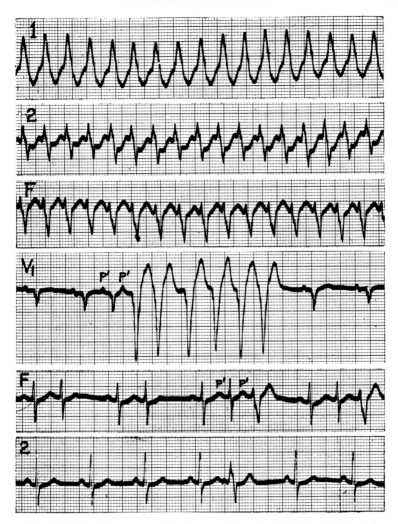

FIG. 145. The three upper strips show a pattern typical of ventricular tachycardia. The lower three strips demonstrate that the tachycardia is supraventricular
with ventricular aberration; the fourth strip shows the beginning of a paroxysm,
which again looks ventricular but which is preceded by the onset of rapid ectopic
atrial activity (P'), indicating that this paroxysm is probably ectopic atrial with
aberrant ventricular conduction. The bottom two strips each show telltale extrasystoles. In lead 2 (bottom strip) there is one bizarre premature beat, which is preceded by an ectopic P wave and followed by a pause that is less than compensa-

Legend concludes on opposite page

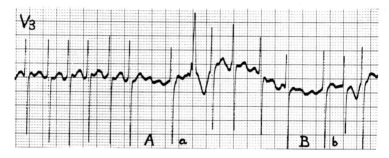

FIG. 146. **Atrial flutter-fibrillation** with **aberrant ventricular conduction.** The rapid ventricular response is interrupted on two occasions by longer-than-usual diastoles (A and B). These long cycles lengthen the ensuing refractory periods of the conducting tissues. After pause A, therefore, the next short cycle, a, is terminated by a distorted (aberrant) ventricular complex of RBBB form. Pause B is not so long as A and produces less prolongation of the refractory period; the beat terminating the ensuing pause b shows only minor signs of aberration —its T wave is deeply inverted and the QRS has decidely lower voltage than any of the other beats.

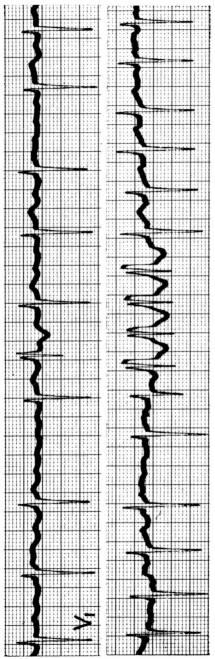

FIG. 147. **Atrial fibrillation** with **aberrant ventricular conduction.** In the upper strip the fifth beat might well be mistaken for an ectopic ventricular beat; however, it terminates a short cycle preceded by a long cycle, is of RBBB form and is more likely an aberrant complex. In the lower strip the fifth beat, which terminates a long diastole, is followed by five aberrant complexes; the first of these shows only minor distortion (slurred upstroke, less deep S wave and frankly inverted T wave) but the following four beats show gross RBBB, which could readily be mistaken for a short burst of ventricular tachycardia.

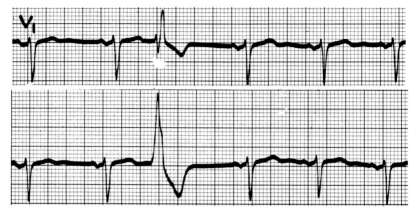

FIG. 148. Two strips of V_1 from the same patient. The upper strip shows an atrial premature beat with ventricular aberration; the lower strip, a ventricular premature beat. Note that the aberrant beat has an initial deflection identical with those of the flanking sinus beats and a triphasic (rsR′) contour, whereas the ectopic ventricular beat is monophasic (R). (Reproduced from Sandler and Marriott: The differential morphology of anomalous ventricular complexes of RBBB-type in lead V_1. Circulation 1965: 31, 551.)

It is often difficult and sometimes impossible to distinguish aberration from ventricular ectopy by the morphology of the anomalous complexes. But when the anomalous complexes are upright in V_1, i.e., giving a RBBB pattern, there are a few helpful pointers.

Since 80 per cent of aberrant beats are of RBBB form (20) and presumably represent a type of RBBB, and since the development of RBBB usually leaves the initial QRS forces undisturbed, aberration of this type should show an initial vector identical with that of flanking conducted beats. Surprisingly, only 44 per cent of 50 aberrant patterns lived up to this expectation—presumably because there was often an associated conduction delay on the left side, perhaps a hemiblock.

Secondly, about 70 per cent of aberrant beats show a triphasic $+ - +$ (usually rsR′) pattern in V_1, the rest having a monophasic (R) or diphasic (qR) pattern. More important, beats that fulfil all the conventional criteria for ventricular premature beats almost *never* show an RSR′ pattern and almost *always* have an initial deflection that differs from that of the flanking conducted beats. Therefore, if the beat in V_1 (or another right

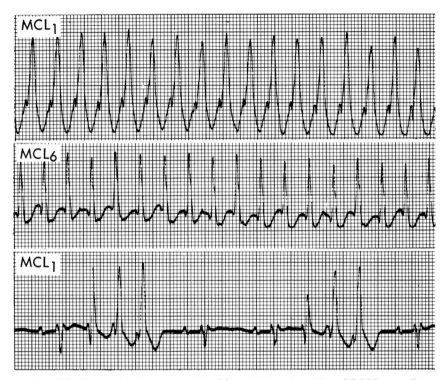

FIG. 149. **Supraventricular tachycardia** with **ventricular aberration** of RBBB type. From the top strip of MCL_1, one cannot differentiate between left ventricular tachycardia and supraventricular tachycardia with RBBB-type aberration; but the qRs pattern in MCL_6 strongly favors a supraventricular mechanism. In the bottom strip, the rsR' pattern of the first beat of each burst confirms the supraventricular origin.

chest lead such as MCL_1) shows an RSR' pattern, the odds are heavily in favor of aberration; and if it shows an identical initial deflection as well, the odds are overwhelmingly for aberration. Figure 148 illustrates a typical ventricular premature beat and an aberrantly conducted atrial premature beat compared in the same tracing. Lead V_6 (or MCL_6) is equally helpful in that it generally shows a reciprocally triphasic $- + -$ (usually qRs) pattern, and this may look obviously "supraventricular" (fig. 149) even when V_1 (or MCL_1) shows one of the less characteristic forms (R or qR).

** ALL THAT'S ANOMALOUS ISN'T ECTOPIC **

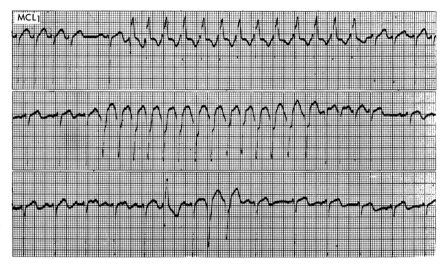

FIG. 150. Runs of atrial tachycardia with **aberrant conduction** of RBBB type in top strip and of LBBB type in 2nd strip. Both forms are present in bottom strip.

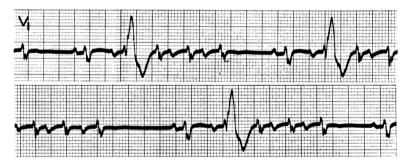

FIG. 151. The second beat in each group shows **ventricular aberration** of RBBB type.

The Hallmarks of Aberration

1. Preceding P' wave
2. RBBB pattern
3. Triphasic contour in lead V_1 (rsR') and V_6 (qRs)
4. Initial vector identical with that of flanking conducted beats
5. Second in a group

It is not at all uncommon to see both RBBB and LBBB aberration follow each other in quick succession in the same tracing (fig. 150).

Another clue: when *only the second* in a group of rapid beats shows an anomalous pattern (fig. 151), you can be almost sure that it is aberrant and not ectopic. This is because such a beat is the only beat that ends a relatively short cycle preceded by a relatively long cycle. All the other beats either end short cycles preceded by short cycles, or end long cycles. The five most helpful criteria for recognizing aberration are summarized below, and they are all evident in the anomalous beats in figure 151.

In the presence of atrial fibrillation, the responsible atrial impulse is of course not recognizable, and we must lean heavily on morphologic clues and other criteria (14).

DIFFERENTIATION BETWEEN SUPRAVENTRICULAR AND VENTRICULAR TACHYCARDIAS (16, 18)

With close attention to clinical detail, the bedside diagnosis of regular tachycardia can be surprisingly accurate. First some principles, misconceptions and false doctrines:

1. The proper posture for the diagnostician at the bedside is to apply stethoscope to the precordium and eyes to the neck veins *simultaneously*.
2. Clues to search for are:
   a. Presence or absence of cannon "a" waves or flutter waves in the jugular pulse.
   b. Variation in intensity of the first heart sound.
   c. Splitting of the heart sounds.
3. Splitting of the sounds is due to ventricular *asynchrony*, whereas *irregular* cannon waves in the neck and variation in intensity of the first sound are signs of *dissociation* between atria and ventricles.
4. Signs of dissociation are more easily identified at the bedside than in the tracing because the independent P waves are more often than not lost in the barrage of ventricular complexes.
5. *Dissociation does not prove ventricular tachycardia;* but it excludes atrial trachycardia and therefore makes ventricular that much more likely. Dissociation can occur between atrial and A-V pacemakers and, if ventricular aberration is also present, the imitation of ventricular tachycardia may be perfect both clinically and electrocardiographically.
6. *Regular* cannon waves—with every beat—may be seen in atrial tachycardia, A-V tachycardia or ventricular tachycardia with 1:1 retroconduction.

The *electrocardiographic* recognition of typical supraventricular tachycardia is easy; the difficulty arises in separating ventricular tachycardia from a supraventricular tachycardia combined with ventricular aberration. Although the demonstration of dissociation is of limited diagnostic value, evidence of it should always be sought. If P waves are not recognizable even in V_1, more specialized leads may be informative: a precordial lead taken from an interspace above V_1 (atrial lead point; see fig. 2, page 2) may reveal P waves, and for this the CR connection may be more useful than the V. If this is unsuccessful, a lead known as S_5 may be tried (10): for this the positive electrode is placed in the 5th right interspace close to the sternal border and the negative electrode over the manubrium (with the conventional patient cable, the LA electrode is placed in the 5th interspace with the RA electrode on the manubrium, and the selector switch is set for standard lead 1.) If this fails, an esophageal (3, 7) or intracardiac (23) lead will almost always be successful in displaying P waves. Alternatively, if a tracing is taken during the administration of procaine amide (1) or acetylcholine (21) intravenously, the ventricular rate will often slow under their influence, and P waves will become apparent in the now lengthened intervals between ventricular complexes.

With these many principles in mind, we can formulate a systematic approach to the regular tachycardia:

1. *First look at the neck veins and listen to the first heart sound with the patient holding his breath.* If there are irregular cannon waves in the neck and/or the first heart sound varies in intensity from beat to beat, you have evidence of dissociation, and this suggests a ventricular tachycardia. If the first heart sound is of unvarying intensity and there are either no cannon waves or regular cannon waves in the neck, this is against dissociation and the tachycardia is probably supraventricular (exceptions: a) ventricular tachycardia with retrograde 1:1 conduction; b) ventricular tachycardia with concurrent atrial fibrillation).

    If an electrocardiogram is available, do not use carotid sinus or other vagal stimulation until after one has been taken, because if the tachycardia is supraventricular, the vagal maneuver may terminate it, leaving no graphic record to document the paroxysm.

2. *Take an electrocardiogram* and look at the QRS pattern. If it is normal in contour and duration, the tachycardia is supraventricular. If it is widened and bizarre, the tachycardia may be either ventricular or supraventricular with aberrant ventricular conduction. If it is widened, study the V_1/V_6 morphology. Try to find a lead in which P waves are identifiable and look for Dressler beats. If previous tracings are available, look for isolated extrasystoles and compare their pattern with that of the tachycardia.

3. If the diagnosis is still in doubt, *try carotid sinus stimulation, eyeball compression or other vagal stimulation.* If the tachycardia is supraventricular, this may terminate it. If it is ventricular it will be unaffected. In atrial flutter vagal stimulation may temporarily halve the rate by increasing the A-V conduction ratio from 2:1 to 4:1.

4. If there is still doubt, consider passing an *esophageal* or *intracardiac electrode*; a satisfactory esophageal or intracardiac lead will always reveal P waves when they are unidentifiable in conventional leads. However, in practice, these invasive techniques are almost never needed and should certainly be avoided whenever possible, especially in patients with acute myocardial infarction.

5. If doubt remains, one may administer *procaine amide intravenously* with appropriate precautions. If the tachycardia is ventricular, this will be a correct treatment; if it is supraventricular, the drug may momentarily block A-V conduction and reveal the telltale atrial rhythm between the now more widely spaced ventricular complexes (1). *Acetylcholine* may have a similar effect (20).

6. If facilities for recording *His-bundle electrograms* are at hand and the clinical circumstances warrant the procedure, this technique may provide the only certain means of differentiating ventricular aberration from ectopy (4).

In summary:

Clinically
1. Look for
    a. Wide splitting of heart sounds.
    b. Variation in intensity of first sound.
    c. Cannon waves.
2. Observe effect of carotid sinus stimulation.

Electrocardiographically (in records that look like ventricular tachycardia):
1. Study the QRS morphology.
2. Identify P waves.
    a. In conventional leads, especially 2 and V_1.
    b. In lead S_5.
    c. In esophageal or intracardiac lead.
    d. During administration of procaine amide or acetylcholine.
3. Look for Dressler beats.
4. Look for isolated extrasystoles in previous tracings.

REFERENCES

1. Bernstein, L. M., et al.: Intravenous procaine amide as an aid to differentiate flutter with bundle branch block from paroxysmal ventricular tachycardia. Am. Heart J. 1954: **48**, 82.

2. Cohen, S. I., et al.: Variations of aberrant ventricular conduction in man. Circulation 1968: **38**, 899.

3. Copeland, G. D., et al.: Clinical evaluation of a new esophageal electrode, with particular reference to the bipolar esophageal electrocardiogram. Part II. Observations in cardiac arrhythmias. Am. Heart J. 1959: **57**, 874.

4. Damato, A. N., and Lau, S. H.: Clinical value of the electrogram of the conduction system. Prog. Cardiovasc. Dis. 1970: **13**, 119.

5. Gouaux, J. L., and Ashman, R.: Auricular fibrillation with aberration simulating ventricular paroxysmal tachycardia. Am. Heart J. 1947: **34**, 366.

6. Kistin, A. D.; Retrograde conduction to the atria in venticular tachycardia. Circulation 1961: **24**, 236.

7. Kistin, A. D.: Problems in the differentiation of ventricular arrhythmia from supraventricular arrhythmia with abnormal QRS. Progr. Cardiovasc. Dis. 1966: **9**, 1.

8. Langendorf, R.: Differential diagnosis of ventricular paroxysmal tachycardia. Exper. Med. Surg. 1950: **8**, 228.

9. Langendorf, R.: Aberrant ventricular conduction. Am. Heart J 1951: **41**, 700.

10. Lian, Cassimatis and Hebert: Intéret de la dérivation précordiale auriculaire S₅ dans le diagnostic des troubles du rythme auriculaire. Arch. Mal. Coeur 1952: **45**, 481.

11. Marriott, H. J. L.: Things aren't always what they seem. Current Med. Digest 1958: **25**, No. 8 (August), 60; ibid. 1958: **25**, No. 11 (November), 70; ibid. 1959: **26**, No. 2 (February), 79.

12. Marriott, H. J. L., and Schamroth, L.: Important dilemmas in cardiac arrhythmias. Maryland State Med. J. 1959: **8**, 660.

13. Marriott, H. J. L.: Simulation of ectopic ventricular rhythms by aberrant conduction. J.A.M.A. 1966: **196**, 787.

14. Marriott, H. J. L., and Sandler, I. A.: Criteria, old and new, for differentiating between ectopic ventricular beats and aberrant ventricular conduction in the presence of atrial fibrillation. Progr. Cardiovasc. Dis. 1966: **9**, 18.

15. Marriott, H. J. L., and Menendez, M. M.: A-V dissociation revisited. Progr. Cardiovasc. Dis. 1966: **8**, 522.

16. Marriott, H. J. L.: Differential diagnosis of supraventricular and ventricular tachycardia. Geriatrics 1970: **25**, 91.

17. Marriott, H. J. L., and Thorne, D. C.: Dysrhythmic dilemmas in coronary care. Am. J. Cardiol. 1971: **27**, 327.

18. Pick, A., and Langendorf, R.: Differentiation of supraventricular and ventricular tachycardias. Progr. Cardiovasc. Dis. 1960: **2**, 391.

19. Rubin, I. L., et al.: The esophageal lead in the diagnosis of tachycardias with aberrant ventricular conduction. Am. Heart J. 1959: **57**, 19.

20. Sandler, I. A., and Marriott, H. J. L.: The differential morphology of anomalous ventricular complexes of RBBB-type in lead V₁: ventricular ectopy versus aberration. Circulation 1965: **31**, 551.

21. Schoolman, H. M., et al.: Acetylcholine in differential diagnosis and treatment of paroxysmal tachycardia. Am. Heart J. 1960: **60**, 526.

22. Schrire, V., and Vogelpoel, L.: The clinical and electrocardiographic differentiation of supraventricular and ventricular tachycardias with regular rhythm. Am. Heart J. 1955: **49**, 162.

23. Vogel, J. H. K., et al.: A simple technique for identifying **P** waves in complex arrhythmias. Am. Heart J. 1964: **67**, 158.

Review Tracings

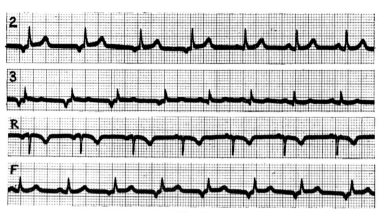

TR-10

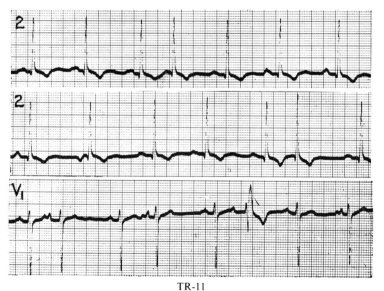

TR-11

For interpretations, see pages 314–17

Review Tracing

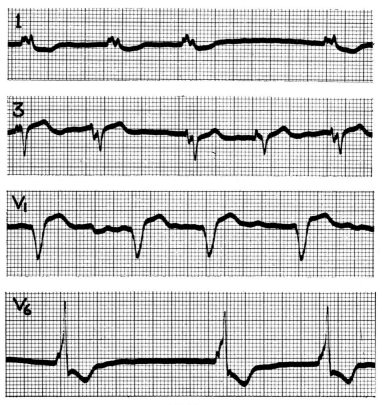

TR-12
For interpretation, see pages 314–17

14

The Wolff-Parkinson-White Syndrome

This purely electrocardiographic "syndrome" (16) bears a superficial resemblance to bundle-branch block and has therefore sometimes been called "pseudo-BBB." But with the common denominator of a widened QRS complex, the similarity ends.

If the pattern of bundle-branch block is superimposed on a normal P-QRS sequence, we get the composite picture indicated in figure 152A; the blocked ventricle is activated late so that the superadded deflection is tacked on to the end of the normal QRS, leaving the P-R interval untouched. In the W-P-W syndrome the superadded deflection is attached in front of the normal QRS, thus shortening the P-R interval by as much as it lengthens the QRS (fig. 152B). In bundle-branch block the QRS is pro-

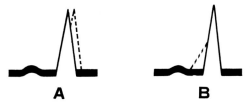

| A | B |

Fig. 152. A. Bundle-branch block and B. Wolff-Parkinson-White syndrome compared diagrammatically.

longed because one ventricle is activated late; the W-P-W syndrome results when one ventricle (or part of a ventricle) is activated abnormally early (**pre-excitation**).

This explanation is generally accepted, but the exact mechanism of early activation of one ventricle is in dispute. It is widely believed that accelerated conduction to one ventricle is effected through an accessory bundle (bundle of Kent) which bypasses the A-V node and bundle and so avoids the pause which normally occurs when the impulse arrives at the A-V junctional tissues. Accessory bundles are generally thought of as bridging the atrioventricular groove at the free wall of the right ventricle; but there is no doubt that the accessory tracts can be more centrally located and bypass fibers close to the A-V junction have been identified and incriminated (7, 9).

Prinzmetal et al. (13) gave evidence that the asynchronous activation of the ventricles in this "syndrome" is due to differential transmission of the impulse at the A-V node itself—that most of the impulse suffers its normal delay at the A-V node, while part of the impulse speeds ahead to its ventricular destination. They suggested **accelerated conduction syndrome** as a descriptive alternative for Wolff-Parkinson-White syndrome. Sherf and James (15) postulate an ectopic focus in the posterior internodal tract with a disturbed pattern of conduction through the A-V junction and consequent asymmetrical arrival of impulses within the ventricles.

The classical pattern consists of a shortened P-R interval followed by a lengthened QRS interval. The QRS is as much longer than normal as the P-R interval is shorter than normal. The P-R interval usually measures 0.10 sec. or less, and the P wave is normal. The initial deflection of the QRS is slurred, producing the so-called delta wave (fig. 153).

The pattern, however, is not always so typical. Sometimes the P-R interval may not be frankly shortened, or the QRS may not be prolonged above the limits of normal; yet a telltale delta wave may indicate the true mechanism.

Patterns of the W-P-W syndrome have been variously classified. In 1945 Rosenbaum and Wilson divided them into two groups, A and B. Group A had predominantly positive ventricular complexes in V_1 (fig. 153), whereas

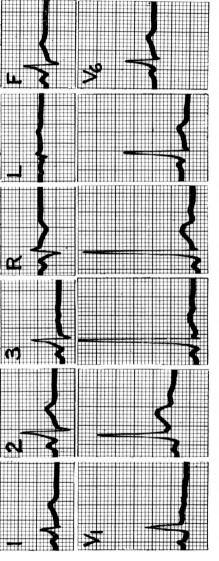

FIG. 153. **Wolff-Parkinson-White syndrome.** Note short P-R intervals (0.10 sec.) and wide QRS complexes with slurred upstrokes in leads 1, 2, 3, aVF and V_{2-6}.

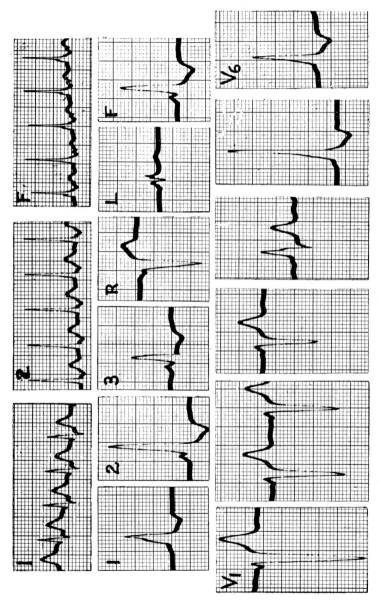

FIG. 154. **Wolff-Parkinson-White syndrome.** Note short P-R interval and wide QRS complexes with delta waves (slurred initial upstrokes), especially in leads 1 and V_{5-6}. The tendency to paroxysmal tachycardia is indicated in the top row, where a supraventricular tachycardia at rate 165 is displayed.

group B complexes in V₁ were predominantly negative (fig. 154). Grant (3) pointed out that this differentiation was based on a relatively insignificant shift of the ventricular vector and introduced a new classification based on the axis of the delta wave in the frontal plane: type I—the commonest— had a delta-wave axis in the neighborhood of −30° and so produced Q waves in leads, 2, 3 and a VF stimulating inferior infarction (fig. 155). Type III—the least common—had a delta-wave axis of about +105° and so produced small wide Q waves in leads 1 and aVL simulating anterior or lateral infarction. Type II had an axis between the other two, at about +50°. There seems to be little practical value in either classification, but that most commonly employed is "type A" and "type B," corresponding with Wilson's groups A and B.

This syndrome is relatively benign. It predominantly affects males and is found in all age groups. In the younger subjects, it occurs mainly in individuals with no sign of heart disease; however, it is found in a significant

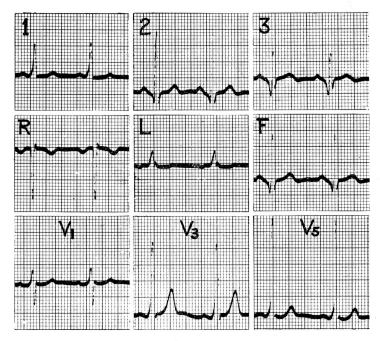

Fig. 155. **Wolff-Parkinson-White syndrome,** showing atypical features: the P-R interval is normal at 0.16 sec., the QRS slightly prolonged at 0.10 to 0.11 sec. Delta waves are clearly seen in leads 1, V₃ and V₅. The slurred initial component in leads 2, 3 and aVF takes the form of wide Q waves, which may be mistaken for those of inferior myocardial infarction if the over-all pattern is not recognized.

number of young patients with idiopathic hypertrophic subaortic stenosis and type B W-P-W occurs in 25 per cent of those with Ebstein's disease (13). In many of the older patients, this anomaly of conduction appears to result from serious heart disease and is therefore not always associated with a benign prognosis.

In most patients the only other cardiac peculiarity is a tendency to atrial arrhythmias; and in those with arrhythmias, paroxysmal atrial tachycardia is reported in 70 per cent, atrial fibrillation in 16 per cent, unidentified supraventricular tachycardia in 10 per cent and atrial flutter in 4 per cent (12). In many cases the mechanism of what appears to be atrial tachy-cardia is probably a circulating (or "reentering") wave using both acces-sory (or bypass) bundle and the A-V junction—going down one and up the other (1). Whether the QRS is normal or bizarre during the tachycardia depends on whether the A-V junction or the accessory path is used as the downward limb of the circuit. When the QRS remains wide and bizarre, the W-P-W syndrome is an important mimic of ventricular tachycardia (fig. 156) (11) and many examples of atrial fibrillation with W-P-W conduction have been published erroneously as irregular ventricular tachycardia. Type A W-P-W, with wide upright complexes across the precordium, can be par-ticularly deceptive. One should always be suspicious that a W-P-W is at work when the ventricular rate is unusually rapid—over 240 (5).

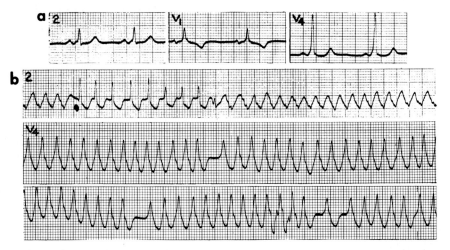

Fig. 156. **a.** Illustrates typical features of **type A W-P-W. b.** Illustrates the wild, irregular tachycardias that can complicate the W-P-W syndrome and be mistaken for ventricular tach-ycardia and even fibrillation ("pseudoventricular" tachycardia and fibrillation).

REFERENCES

1. Durrer, D., et al.: Pre-excitation revisited. Am. J. Cardiol. 1970: **25**, 690.
2. Ferrer, M. I.: New concepts relating to the preexcitation syndrome. JAMA 1967: **201**, 1038.
3. Grant, R. P., et al.: Ventricular activation in the pre-excitation syndrome (Wolff-Parkinson-White). Circulation 1958: **18**, 355.
4. Hejtmancik, M. R., and Herrmann, G. R.: The electrocardiographic syndrome of short P-R interval and broad QRS complexes. A clinical study of 80 cases. Am. Heart J. 1957: **54**, 708.
5. Herrmann, G. R., et al.: Paroxysmal pseudoventricular tachycardia and pseudoventricular fibrillation in patients with accelerated A-V conduction. Am. Heart J. 1957: **53**, 254.
6. James, T. N.: The Wolff-Parkinson-White syndrome. Ann. Int. Med. 1969: **71**, 399.
7. James, T. N.: The Wolff-Parkinson-White syndrome: evolving concepts of its pathogenesis. Progr. Cardiovasc. Dis. 1970: **13**, 159.
8. Kariv, I.: Wolff-Parkinson-White syndrome simulating myocardial infarction. Am. Heart J. 1958: **55**, 406.
9. Lev, M., et al.: Anatomic findings in a case of ventricular pre-excitation (WPW) terminating in complete atrioventricular block. Circulation 1966: **34**, 718.
10. Lown, B., et al.: The syndrome of the short P-R interval, normal QRS complex and paroxysmal rapid heart action. Circulation 1952: **5**, 693.
11. Marriott, H. J. L., and Rogers, H. M.: Mimics of ventricular tachycardia associated with the W-P-W syndrome. J. Electrocardiol. 1969: **2**, 77.
12. Newman, B. J., et al.: Arrhythmias in the Wolff-Parkinson-White syndrome. Prog. Cardiovasc. Dis. 1966: **9**, 147.
13. Prinzmetal, M., et al.: Accelerated conduction. *The Wolff-Parkinson-White Syndrome and Related Conditions.* Grune and Stratton, New York, 1952.
14. Schiebler, G. L., et al.: The Wolff-Parkinson-White syndrome in infants and children. Pediatrics 1959: **24**, 585.
15. Sherf, L., and James, T. N.: A new look at some old questions in clinical electrocardiography. Henry Ford Hosp. Med. Bull. 1966: **14**, 265.
16. Wolff, L.: Syndrome of short P-R interval with abnormal QRS complexes and paroxysmal tachycardia (Wolff-Parkinson-White syndrome). Circulation 1954: **10**, 282.
17. Wolff, L.: Wolff-Parkinson-White syndrome: historical and clinical features. Progr. Cardiovasc. Dis. 1960: **2**, 677.

Review Tracings

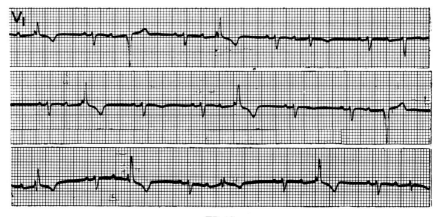

TR-13

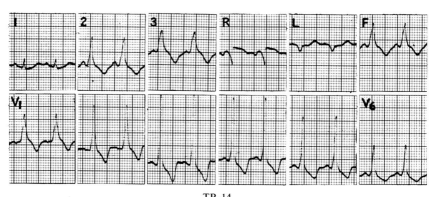

TR-14

For interpretations, see pages 314–17

Review Tracing

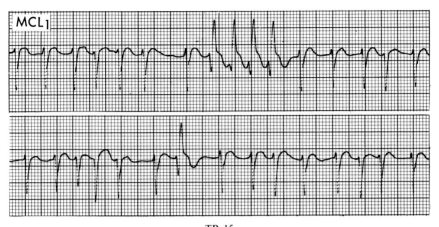

TR-15

For interpretation, see pages 314–17

15

Intra-Atrial, Sino-Atrial, and Atrio-Ventricular Block

INTRA-ATRIAL BLOCK

If the impulse takes longer than normal to activate the atria, i.e., if the P wave is widened, intra-atrial block is said to be present. The upper normal limit of P-wave duration is not universally agreed upon, but the most satisfactory limit is probably 0.11 sec. The criterion, therefore, for diagnosing intra-atrial block is a P wave with a duration of 0.12 sec. or more (fig. 157). Further evidence of block is to be found in deep notching of the P wave with a distance between peaks ("peak interval") of more than 0.04 sec. (fig. 157 C).

Intra-atrial block is not uncommon and is most often seen in coronary disease, mitral disease and in association with left ventricular hypertrophy (1). It probably often represents atrial enlargement rather than true block and is thus analogous to the term intraventricular block applied to the QRS interval of 0.11 sec. or more when this is due to ventricular enlargement.

When the heart actually drops a beat, it means either that the S-A node has failed to initiate the impulse (S-A block) or, much more likely, that the impulse after traversing the atria has been unable to get through the A-V conducting tissues (A-V block). Both these types of block may be recognized in any lead in which P waves are clearly formed.

S-A BLOCK

S-A block is divided into incomplete and complete:

194

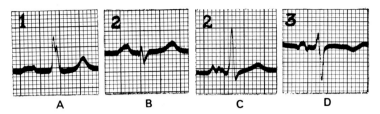

FIG. 157. **Intra-atrial block.** Four samples from four different patients. A and B show widening of P wave without significant notching; C and D show marked notching with wide peak interval (more than 0.04 sec.).

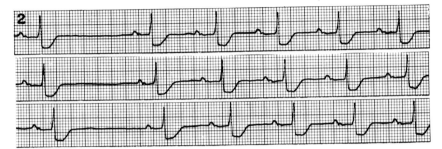

FIG. 158. **Incomplete-S-A block.** The strips are continuous. The long cycle at the beginning of each strip is due to a dropped sinus beat—an entire P-QRS-T sequence is missing.

1. **Incomplete S-A block** consists in the more or less infrequent suppression of impulse formation at, or failure to emerge from, the S-A node, with the result that occasional beats are completely dropped. This is recognized in the tracing by the occasional absence of the entire P-QRS-T sequence (fig. 158 and 159).

2. **Complete S-A block** exists when *no* impulses are formed in, or emerge from, the S-A node and therefore no P waves are inscribed. This situation is also referred to as **atrial paralysis** or **atrial standstill.** But atrial paralysis can also occur in potassium intoxication without S-A block (see p. 304).

In the absence of S-A leadership, one of two things can happen: either a) a lower pacemaker, usually in the A-V junction but sometimes in the ventricles, comes to the rescue and takes over the job of pacemaking, or b) cardiac standstill continues and the patient dies. If a) occurs and the ventricles proceed to beat independently, **nodal** or **ventricular escape** is said to

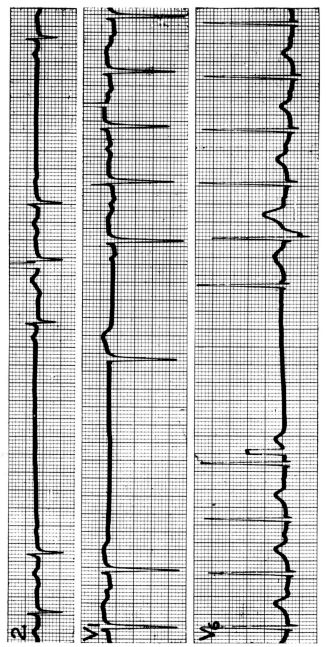

FIG. 159. Runs of sinus rhythm at a rate of about 100 are punctuated by periods of S-A block. Two such periods occur in lead 2. In V_1 the period of atrial standstill is terminated by an **A-V nodal escape beat**. In V_6 a similar pause is terminated by an escape beat which is followed by a run of sinus rhythm, the first beat of which shows **ventricular aberration**.

have occurred and the heart's rhythm is called idionodal or idioventricular. Complete S-A block is thus one of the two mechanisms (much the less common) leading to the development of **idioventricular rhythm.**

Complete S-A block is recognized in the electrocardiogram by the complete absence of the entire P-QRS-T sequence, i.e., by a straight and unadorned baseline; this continues until, if the patient is fortunate, independent QRST complexes appear at a slow rate while P waves remain absent.

S-A block is rather rare, but it can be produced by a wide variety of causes: *drugs*, such as digitalis, quinidine and salicylates; *diseases*, such as coronary disease and acute infections; *physiological* disturbances, such as carotid sinus sensitivity and increased vagal tone.

Salient Features of S-A Block

1. Incomplete: occasional absence of P-QRS-T sequence
2. Complete:
   a. P waves absent
   b. QRST sequence at slow rate
   c. QRS interval normal or prolonged, depending on site of ventricular pacemaker

---

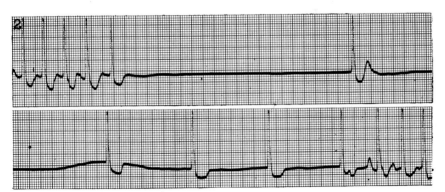

Fig. 160. "**Sick sinus syndrome.**" Irregular atrial tachycardia followed by a prolonged sinus pause punctuated by all too few, badly needed A-V escape beats.

SICK SINUS SYNDROME

In some patients, bursts of an atrial tachyarrhythmia—often fibrillation —alternate with prolonged periods of sinus arrest (fig. 160). In such cases, the sinus node is abnormally susceptible to the suppressive influence of the ectopic atrial activity and remains quiescent for uncomfortably long periods. This situation is refractory to therapy and has sometimes been called "sick sinus syndrome" (9) and sometimes "tachycardia-bradycardia syndrome" (2, 11). Some authorities include any form of marked sinus nodal depression (marked sinus bradycardia, S-A block), with or without the intermittent tachyarrhythmia, under the heading of sick sinus syndrome.

A-V BLOCK

Several important points should be made about the subject of A-V block in general before delving into the details of specific types. First of all, block is an *abnormal* delay or failure of conduction and it must be kept distinct from *normal* delay or failure due to physiological refractoriness. For example, when the fluttering atria beat at a rate of 320 per minute, it is healthy, desirable refractoriness of the A-V conducting tissues that protects the ventricles and prevents them from receiving every impulse. Atrial flutter with 2 to 1 conduction is a more accurate term than 2 to 1 block.

Next, remember that you cannot diagnose block unless there was adequate *opportunity* for conduction. For example, if an accelerated idioventricular rhythm develops (see page 116) and usurps control from the sinus node at a slightly faster rate, the lower pacemaker may remain dissociated from the higher for several cycles—with P waves trailing just behind the QRS with no chance of conduction to the ventricles. This is dissociation, yes, but not block. And this introduces the third point: that block and dissociation are not by any means synonymous. A-V dissociation may be due to many causes—of which block is but one (see page 213). All three of these points highlight the aphorism: absence of conduction is not the same as block.

Finally, one should keep in mind that our definitions of the various divisions and degrees of block are only *relatively* accurate. This is because the significance of block must always be assessed in the light of attendant circumstances—the most important of which is the heart rate. Thus, 4 to 1

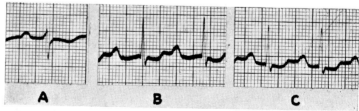

FIG. 161. **1st degree A-V block.** The P-R interval is prolonged. A. P-R interval is 0.26 sec. B. P-R interval is 0.34 sec. and in this case is caused by digitalis. C. Same patient as B, showing effect of forced inspiration: note increase in rate and decrease in P-R interval to 0.22 sec.

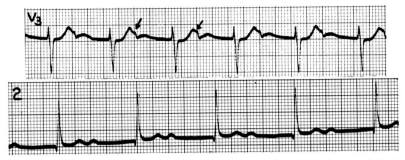

FIG. 162. Two examples of **1st degree A-V block.** In the upper strip two of the P waves are indicated by arrows and the P-R interval is about 0.46 sec. In the bottom strip the P-R is about 0.59 sec.

conduction when the atria are fluttering at a rate of 300 is a satisfactory state of affairs and represents relatively unimportant block; this is in stark contrast with 4 to 1 conduction when the atrial rate is 80. Again the implications are far different if the atria, at a rate of 70, are dissociated from ventricles beating at 80 than if they were dissociated from an idioventricular rhythm at a rate of 30. Yet our definitions for block seldom give the heart rate and other attendant circumstances the consideration that is their due.

Classification of A-V block

A-V block is also divided into incomplete and complete; first and second degrees of A-V block are forms of incomplete block, whereas third degree is the same as complete block. In mild disturbances of A-V conduction, the impulse merely takes longer to travel from atria to ventricles—it is delayed in the A-V junction and A-V conduction time (P-R interval) is prolonged—first degree A-V block (figs. 161 and 162). In severer grades of block the atrial impulse is at times held up at the A-V node or bundle, or in both bundle branches simultaneously, fails to reach the ventricles and a "dropped beat" results. When beats are dropped, second degree A-V block is established which is recognized in the tracing by the presence of isolated P waves not followed by ventricular complexes (figs. 163–168).

Second degree A-V block requires further subdivision. In 1899, Wenckebach in Vienna observed dropped beats in a jugular pulse tracing; and he noted that the dropped beat was preceded by progressive prolongation of the interval between atrial and ventricular contraction. Wenckebach again in 1906, once more without benefit of electrocardiogram, observed dropped beats preceded by constant A-V conduction intervals; and Hay, in Scotland, in the same year independently made the same observation. It was nearly twenty years later that Mobitz proposed that these two forms of incomplete A-V block be called type I and type II respectively.

Type I A-V block (Wenckebach phenomenon)

Type I A-V block is relatively benign. The block occurs high in the A-V junction (3) and is usually associated with acute reversible conditions (inferior myocardial infarction, rheumatic fever or digitalis intoxication). It is therefore usually a transient disturbance and seldom progresses to complete block.

The Wenckebach phenomenon

The P-R interval may begin within normal limits or it may be somewhat prolonged; then with each successive beat the P-R interval gradually lengthens until finally an impulse fails to reach the ventricles and a beat is dropped. Following the dropped beat the P-R interval reverts to normal, or near normal, and the sequence is repeated. At times the P-R interval may stretch to surprising lengths; in figure 164, for example, one P-R measures 0.80 sec.

Progressive lengthening of the P-R interval occurs because each successive beat arrives earlier and earlier in the relative refractory period of the A-V junction and therefore takes longer to penetrate and reach the ventricles. In tachycardias it may be a physiological mechanism, but at normal rates it implies definite impairment of A-V conduction although it has been rarely reported in apparently normal hearts. The progressive lengthening usually follows a predictable pattern: the maximal increment of one P-R over its predecessor develops between the first and second cycles and in subsequent cycles the increment is less and less. This in turn leaves its mark on the rhythm of the ventricles: following the pause of the dropped beat, the R-R intervals tend to shorten (fig. 163); and the long cycle (containing the dropped beat) is always less than two of the shorter cycles—because it contains the shortest P-R interval. Recognition of this pattern sometimes enables one to spot the phenomenon in action even when there

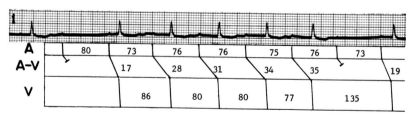

Fig. 163. **Wenckebach phenomenon.** Figures indicate intervals in hundredths of a second. The P-R intervals progressively lengthen until a beat is dropped. Note that the biggest increment (11) is in the second P-R (28) over the first (17) and that there is a tendency for the increments to become less and less (11–3–3–1). The effect of this is to cause progressive shortening of the ventricular cycles 86–80–80–77). (Reproduced from Marriott: *Armchair Arrhythmias*. Tampa Tracings, 1965.)

are no P-R intervals available to measure. Looking back, one can now see that this is the type of sinus block in figure 158: careful measurement shows that the P wave is dropped after a series of gradually shortening P-P intervals, and that the pause of the dropped beat is equal to slightly less than two of the shorter cycles. Another example is seen in fig. 165.

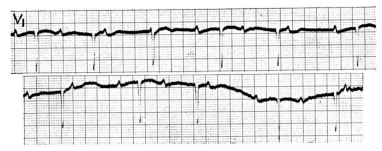

FIG. 164. **Wenckebach phenomenon** with unusually long P-R prolongation. The strips are continuous and display four brief Wenckebach periods; most of these consist merely of two lengthening P-R intervals followed by a dropped beat. At the beginning of the upper strip, however, the three lengthening P-R intervals measure 0.32, 0.55 and 0.80 sec., respectively.

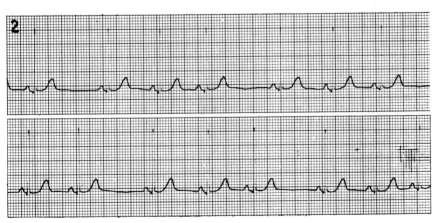

FIG. 165. **Sinus Wenckebach periods** from an 8-year-old boy with a streptococcal tonsillitis. Notice that the sinus cycles show a regularly repeated sequence—progressively shortening cycles leaving the beats grouped in trios. These therefore represent 4:3 sinus Wenckebach periods.

** LEARN TO RECOGNIZE WENCKEBACH BY HIS FOOTPRINTS RATHER THAN HIS FACE**

Another clue that alerts one to an underlying Wenckebach mechanism, especially during tachycardia, is the presence of pairs or small groups of beats (figs. 166 and 167 A); this is thanks to the common occurrence of short (3:2, 4:3, etc.) Wenckebach periods. Short Wenckebach periods also often alternate with 2:1 conduction (fig. 167 B).

Type II A-V Block

This much less common form of second degree block is also much more serious. It is usually associated with a BBB pattern and the site of the block is usually below the bundle of His; i.e., in the presence of BBB, the dropped beats are due to intermittent block in the other bundle branch (3). Type II block is therefore a form of bilateral BBB and it usually progresses to complete A-V block with Adams-Stokes seizures. It is recognized when at least two consecutive beats are conducted with the same P-R interval before the dropped beat (fig. 168 A).

Notice praticularly that you cannot distinguish between type I and type II if only 2:1 conduction is available for study. Both type I and type II can present 2:1 conduction ratios and they can only be distinguished by the company they keep. In figure 167 the 2:1 block in the bottom strip is clearly type I block, because it is sandwiched between Wenckebach periods and the QRS complexes are normally narrow; on the other hand, the 2:1 block in figure 168 is as certainly type II, because the third atrial impulse is blocked after two were conducted with identical P-R intervals, *and* the conducted beats have a BBB pattern.

High grade A-V block

When, at normal atrial rates and in the absence of an accelerated ventricular pacemaker, less than half of the atrial impulses reach the ventricles, advanced or "high-grade" A-V block is present. Perhaps surprisingly, in the presence of such block it is commoner for the beats that are conducted to have normal (figs. 168 A and 169) than prolonged (fig. 168 B) P-R intervals.

Complete A-V block. When *no* impulses can pass the A-V barrier, complete A-V block has developed. Bilateral bundle-branch block, or trifascicular block, rather than blockade at the A-V node or in the main bundle, is often the cause of complete A-V block (7, 8). As with the less common complete S-A block two possibilities now exist. Either the ventricles remain inactive (**ventricular standstill**) and the patient dies, or, more likely, the A-V node (or a lower pacemaker) takes over and controls the ventricles (**nodal** or **ventricular escape**). In this event the atria continue to beat in their own time, and the ventricles beat in a slower tempo, **idioventricular**

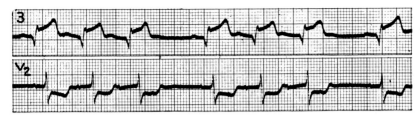

FIG. 166. Sinus tachycardia with 4:3 **Wenckebach periods** which result in the beats being grouped in threes (trigeminy).

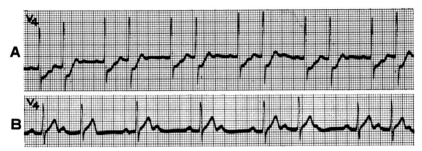

FIG. 167. A. Sinus tachycardia with 3:2 **Wenckebach periods** which result in the beats being grouped in pairs (bigeminy). B. Sinus tachycardia with 3:2 **Wenckebach periods** separated by an intervening run of 2:1 A-V block.

** ALL THAT'S BIGEMINAL ISN'T EXTRASYSTOLIC **

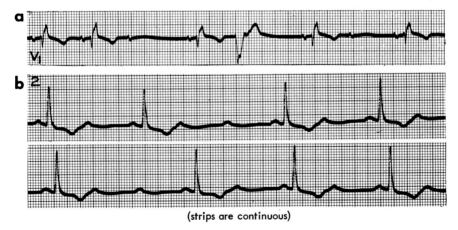

(strips are continuous)

FIG. 168. A. **Second degree A-V block, type II.** Two consecutive P-R intervals are unchanged before the dropped beat. The conducted beats have a normal P-R interval and show RBBB; the 4th beat is a right ventricular premature beat. B. **High grade A-V block.** Sinus rhythm with 2:1 and 3:1 A-V block.

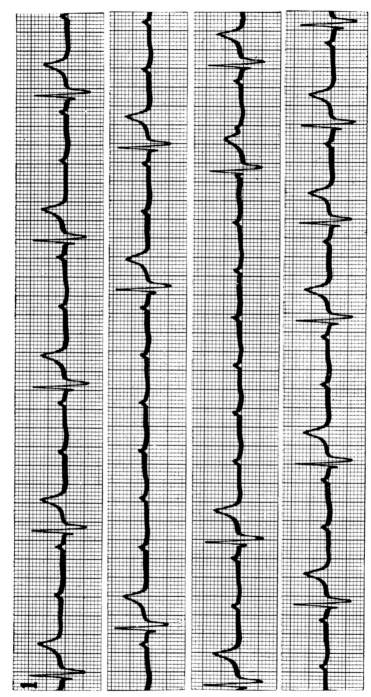

Fig. 169. **High grade A-V block** (the four strips are continuous). 3:1 block is present in the top strip. The second strip contains a 7:1 period. A slightly longer period of ventricular standstill in the third strip is terminated by a nodal escape beat. In the bottom strip there is 3:1 and 2:1 block. Shallow T_p waves are clearly visible following each of the non-conducted P waves.

rhythm. For example, the atria may continue to beat at a sinus rate of 96, while the ventricles perform at 28 (fig. 170). This independence is readily recognized in the tracing by the lack of relationship between the slow ventricular complexes and the more frequent P waves. Each maintains its own rhythm without regard for the other, except that at times *retrograde* conduction to the atria may be seen (fig. 171).

If the idioventricular rhythm is initiated in the A-V junction, the QRS interval and complex will be normal (unless there is concomitant BBB) and the term **idionodal** may properly be applied to the rhythm. If the rescuing pacemaker is in the ventricular muscle itself, then the QRST complex is bizarre with prolonged QRS interval and has the form of an ectopic ventricular beat (figs. 170 and 171).

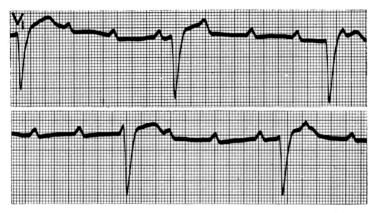

Fɪɢ. 170. **Complete A-V block.** The two strips form a continuous record. P waves and QRS complexes are independent, at ventricular rate of 28, and atrial of 96.

Salient Features of A-V Block

1st degree—prolongation of P-R interval beyond 0.20 sec.
2nd degree—dropped ventricular responses
      Type I—progressive lengthening of P-R intervals until a beat is dropped (Wenckebach phenomenon)
      Type II—consecutively conducted beats with constant P-R intervals before the dropped beat
      High-grade or advanced—two or more consecutively dropped beats (at normal atrial rates)
3rd degree—complete A-V block: no conducted beats in the presence of a slow ventricular rhythm (under 45) and ample opportunity for conduction

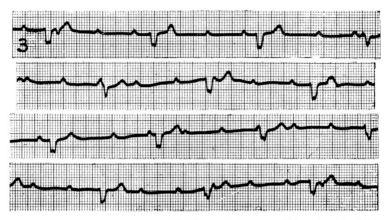

Fig. 171. **Complete A-V block** with idioventricular rate of 36, and atrial of 104. The four strips are continuous. Atrial and ventricular activities are independent except for the first and last ventricular beats—each of these is conducted retrogradely to the atria (note inverted P waves deforming the ST segments of these beats).

Lest there should be any doubt, it is perhaps worth clarifying the difference between idionodal and A-V nodal rhythm. The A-V junction controls the ventricles in both these rhythms. Idionodal rhythm implies that the ventricles have their A-V pacemaker all to themselves and are beating independently of the atria: the atria are either beating in their own time, fibrillating, or they are inactive (complete S-A block). A-V nodal rhythm, on the other hand, means that *both* the ventricles *and* the atria are under A-V control—the A-V junction is the pacemeker of the whole heart.

Complete A-V block is an easy bedside diagnosis. Suspicion is immediately aroused by the slow ventricular rate. Then signs of dissociation between atria and ventricles (variation in intensity of first heart sound with an occasional explosive first sound—"bruit de canon," independent "a" waves and cannon waves in the jugulars, audible independent atrial sounds and sometimes palpable atrial contractions) clinch the diagnosis. Complete block may sometimes be distinguished from 2:1 A-V block by exercise, for this tends to double the rate in 2:1 block but has no effect on the idioventricular rhythm and rate of complete block.

A-V block is often produced by coronary and rheumatic disease varying in incidence with the age group. Less frequently congenital heart disease, cardiomyopathy, syphilis, diphtheria or uremia produces it. Digitalis, quinidine in toxic dosage, procainamide and propranolol (fig. 172) can also induce A-V block. But note that quinidine, lidocaine and diphenylhydantoin can, on occasion, facilitate A-V conduction.

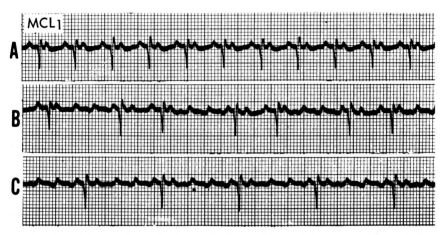

FIG. 172. Illustrates the production of significant A-V block by propranolol. A. Atrial flutter at rate 266 with 2:1 A-V conduction. B. Alternating 2:1 and 4:1 conduction 45 seconds after 2 mg. propranolol i-v. C. 4:1 conduction 2 minutes after propranolol.

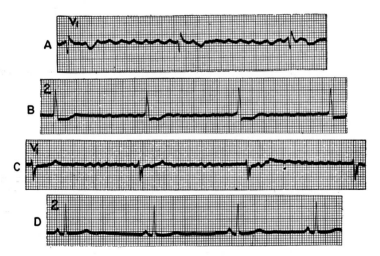

FIG. 173. Various bradycardias. A. **Atrial flutter** with complete A-V block and ventricular rate of 31. B and C. **Atrial fibrillation** with **complete A-V block;** note that ventricular rhythm is absolutely regular, in B at rate 38, in C at 32. D. **Sinus bradycardia** at rate 40–45.

MARKED BRADYCARDIA

As complete A-V block is perhaps the commonest cause of marked bradycardia, it may not be out of place to call attention to other mechanisms. A rate of 30 to 50 may occur in:

1. Idioventricular rhythm—resulting from complete A-V or S-A block (figs. 170, 171)
2. Second degree A-V block—with a sinus rate of, say, 80 and a ventricular rate of 40 (2:1 block)
3. A-V nodal rhythm (fig. 132)
4. Atrial tachycardia (flutter) with high grades of A-V block; e.g., 8:1 block with an atrial rate of 320, giving a ventricular rate of 40
5. Atrial fibrillation with marked A-V block (fig. 173 B and C)
6. Sinus bradycardia (fig. 173 D)

PROLONGED QRS INTERVAL

We can now summarize the conditions associated with a prolonged intraventricular conduction time:

1. When the impulse is initiated in an ectopic ventricular focus
   a. Ventricular premature beat
   b. Ventricular escape beat
   c. Ventricular tachycardia
   d. Idioventricular rhythm (from a low pacemaker)
   e. Accelerated idioventricular rhythm
   f. Ventricular parasystole
   g. Artificial pacemaker
2. When intraventricular conduction is slowed
   a. Intraventricular block
   b. Ventricular aberration
3. When conduction to one ventricle is accelerated
   a. Wolff-Parkinson-White syndrome

REFERENCES

1. Bradley, S. M., and Marriott, H. J. L.: Intra-atrial block. Circulation 1956: **14**, 1073.
2. Cheng, T. O.: Transvenous ventricular pacing in treatment of paroxysmal atrial tachyarrhythmias alternating with sinus bradycardia and standstill. Am. J. Cardiol. 1968: **22**, 874.
3. Damato, A. N., and Lau, S. H.: Clinical value of the electrogram of the conduction system. Prog. Cardiovasc. Dis. 1970: **13**, 119.
4. Johnson, R. L., et al.: Electrocardiographic findings in 67,375 asymptomatic individuals. VII. A-V block. Am. J. Cardiol. 1960: **6**, 153.
5. Katz, L. N., and Pick, A.: *Clinical Electrocardiography. The Arrhythmias*. Lea and Febiger, Philadelphia, 1956.
6. Langendorf, R., and Pick, A.: Atrioventricular block, type II (Mobitz)—its nature and clinical significance. Circulation 1968: **38**, 819.

7. Lenegre, J.: Etiology and pathology of bilateral bundle branch block in relation to complete heart block. Progr. Cardiovasc. Dis. 1964: **6,** 409.

8. Lepeschkin, E.: The electrocardiographic diagnosis of bilateral bundle branch block in relation to heart block. Progr. Cardiovasc. Dis. 1964: **6,** 445.

9. Lown, B. Electrical reversion of atrial fibrillation. Brit. Heart J. 1967: **29,** 469.

10. Schamroth, L., and Dove, E.: The Wenckebach pehnomenon in sinoatrial block. Brit. Heart J. 1966: **28,** 350.

11. Zipes, D. P., et al.: Artificial atrial and ventricular pacing in the treatment of arrhythmias. Ann. Int. Med. 1969: **70,** 885.

Review Tracing

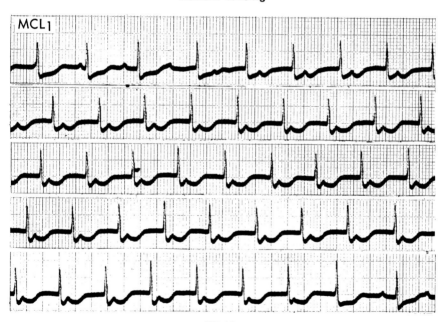

TR-16

For interpretation, see pages 314–17

Review Tracings

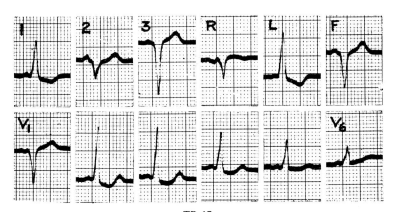

TR-17

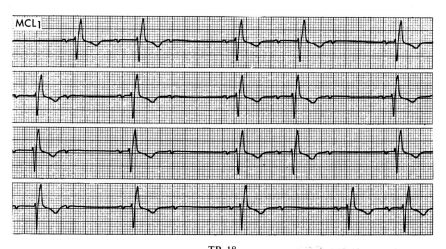

TR-18
For interpretations, see pages 314–17

Some Electrocardiographic Milestones

1858   Kolliker and Muller in Germany demonstrated that contraction of heart muscle was accompanied by electrical activity.

1887   Waller in England recorded the first electrocardiogram in man using a capillary electrometer.

1903   Einthoven in Holland introduced the string galvanometer electrocardiograph and employed the classical standard limb leads in human electrocardiography.

1914   Lewis in England introduced a two-string electrocardiograph. Our knowledge of the sequence of myocardial activation is based on his studies with this machine. Lewis also introduced the concept of the "intrinsic deflection."

1932   Wolferth and Wood in America demonstrated the value of precordial leads.

1934   Wilson in America introduced the central terminal and with it the unipolar or V leads.

1935   Wilson in America demonstrated the superiority of multiple precordial leads over one such lead.

1938   Schellong in Germany and Wilson and Johnston in America described techniques for recording the frontal plane electrocardiogram as a vector figure using the cathode-ray oscillograph.

16

Escape and Dissociation

The dysrhythmic disturbances so far considered have been primary disorders of either impulse formation or conduction. The two phenomena, escape and dissociation, discussed in this chapter, are NOT primary diagnoses—they are, like jaundice or headache, symptomatic of some underlying primary disturbance to which they are secondary.

NODAL AND VENTRICULAR ESCAPE

Escape has been mentioned in connection with both S-A and complete A-V block. It may be regarded as a safety mechanism whereby the heart is rescued when the higher pacemaker fails—the escape beat is indeed "a friend in need." Usually the escaping pacemaker is in the A-V junction **(nodal escape)**, but, if this also defaults, a focus in the ventricles may take over **(ventricular escape)**. Escape may occur for a single beat, ending an unusually long pause, or for but a few beats, or may usher in a more or less permanent idioventricular rhythm. The escape beat is recognized by 1) the absence of a preceding P wave and 2) its *late* appearance, for it occurs only after the next expected beat has failed to appear; it thus ends a longer cycle than the previous R-R intervals. The QRS complexes of nodal escape beats are usually of "supraventricular" form (figs. 174 and 175) whereas ventricular escape beats have the bizarre form of ectopic ventricular beats (fig. 176b). Nodal escape beats, however, quite often show some degree of ventricular aberration (fig. 176a) supposedly because they happen to travel by paraspecific fibers and enter the ventricles via an unorthodox approach (3).

A-V DISSOCIATION

A-V dissociation is used in a number of ways. 1) As a broad, generic

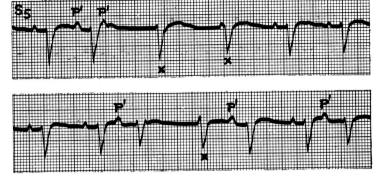

FIG. 174. **Nodal escape.** The two strips are a continuous record of lead S₅.
Dominant rhythm is S-A with several **atrial premature beats** (P'). Following
two of these premature beats, longer than usual R-R intervals are terminated
by nodal escape beats (x).

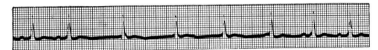

FIG. 175. Transient sinus slowing induced by a deep breath. After the
second beat P waves are suppressed and **A-V nodal escape** occurs for the next
four beats. The S-A node then accelerates and resumes control for the last two
beats.

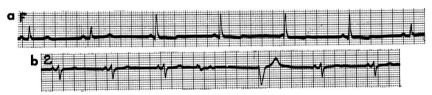

FIG. 176. **Escape beats. a.** Sinus bradycardia with arrhythmia permitting a 4-beat run of
A-V escape with slightly aberrant QRS complexes. **b.** The 4th beat is a VPB and the lengthened postextrasystolic cycle permits a ventricular escape beat to emerge.

term applied to any arrhythmia in which the atria and ventricles beat independently; thus dissociation is momentarily present in a ventricular premature beat and persists during ventricular tachycardia. 2) Complete A-V dissociation has frequently been used as an alternative term for complete A-V
block. 3) In a quasi-specific way it has been applied to the dysrhythmias
whose description follows.

If the excitability of the S-A node becomes unduly depressed, or if the
A-V node becomes unduly excitable, we have seen that the A-V node may

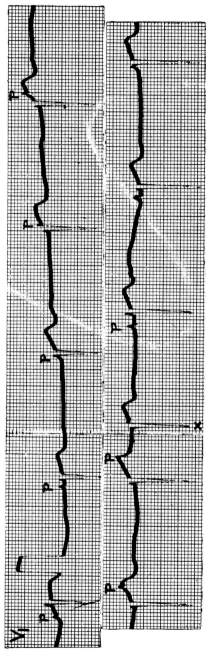

Fig. 177. **A-V dissociation** due to sinus bradycardia. The two strips are a continuous record. The P wave appears first in front of the QRS, but gradually "overtakes" it and by the last beat of the first strip has emerged well beyond the QRS to deform the ST segment. When the P wave falls sufficiently far beyond the QRS (second P in lower strip), the impulse is conducted to the ventricles (third QRS in lower strip). Thus the atria "capture" the ventricles and "interfere" with the otherwise independent ventricular rhythm.

assume control of the heart, producing A-V nodal rhythm. In this rhythm the impulse travels backward into the atria from the A-V node and forward into the ventricles more or less simultaneously. If, however, backward conduction into the atria fails to occur, the atria are protected from A-V nodal control and continue to obey the S-A node, and the stage is set for independent action of atria and ventricles. Thus, in order for this dysrhythmia to develop more than transiently, two fundamentals must be satisfied: 1) the ventricular pacemaker must be firing somewhat faster than the atrial pacemaker, and 2) retrograde conduction must be absent. Forward conduction can still take place, however, so that when the sinus impulse happens to land at a strategic point in the cardiac cycle (when junctional tissues and the ventricles are not refractory), it is conducted to the ventricles (**ventricular capture**). This occasional conducted beat interferes with the rhythm (fig. 177) of the otherwise independent and regularly beating ventricles and has therefore also been called an **interference beat.**

The terminology of this subject has been unnecessarily confused by the experts. The use of the term A-V dissociation for both the dysrhythmias under discussion and complete A-V block—two fundamentally different mechanisms—is the first point of confusion. The second is in the application of the term interference. As used above it refers to the fact that one pacemaker interferes with the rhythm of a second pacemaker. This was the sense implied by Mobitz when he originally introduced the term **interference-dissociation,** and by Scherf when he later modified the term to **dissociation with interference.** Other authorities (1) ignore this use of the term and employ it in an entirely different sense, though a sense no less correct in the terminology of electrophysics. Their "interference" refers to the meeting of two opposing impulses with resulting extinction of both; such interference is seen in fusion beats (page 113) and obviously must occur in A-V dissociation as the independent atrial and ventricular impulses meet, presumably within the A-V junction, and extinguish each other. Thus the "interference" (capture) beat of the first school is the only beat that shows no "interference" of the second type! This paradox is naturally perplexing to the uninitiated, and as neither school ever refers to the perfectly acceptable usage of the other, the confusion is further confounded. Until the terminology of both schools has been grasped, much confusion can be avoided by eschewing the term interference and referring to the conducted beats as capture beats or ventricular captures.

In the electrocardiogram the P waves are seen to "overtake" and pass the QRS complexes (figs. 177 and 178 B). When the P wave falls sufficiently far beyond the QRS, the impulse will be conducted to the ventricles, making them beat prematurely and thus interfering with their otherwise independent rhythm (x in fig. 177). Thus a series of dissociated beats

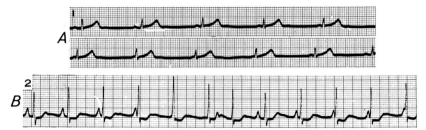

FIG. 178. **A-V dissociation.** In A dissociation results entirely from sinus slowing; in B sinus slowing conspires with enhanced nodal excitability to produce dissociation. The strips in A are continuous and are from a Japanese wrestler, showing how the bradycrotic phase of healthy sinus arrhythmia can lead to A-V nodal escape and A-V dissociation at the normal A-V rate of 46. B is from a 12-year-old girl with digitalis intoxication and severe mitral stenosis. After two normally conducted beats, slight sinus slowing permits the excitable A-V node to escape at a rate of about 78—the P waves "march through" the QRS without hesitating and recapture the ventricles for two beats before dissociation again sets in. (Reproduced from Marriott and Menendez: A-V dissociation revisited. Progr. Cardiovasc. Dis. 1966: **8,** 522.)

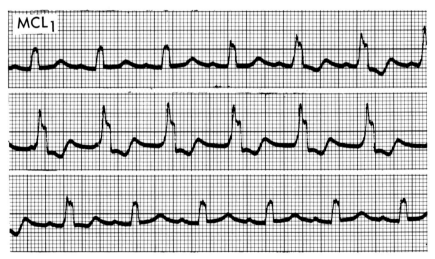

FIG. 179. **A-V dissociation.** Sinus rhythm with RBBB gives place in the top strip to a slightly faster ("usurping") accelerated left idioventricular rhythm; this results in a short run of isorhythmic A-V dissociation with return to sinus rhythm in the bottom strip. The 4th, 5th and 6th beats in top strip and 1st in bottom strip are fusion beats.

** A-V DISSOCIATION, LIKE JAUNDICE, IS A SYMPTOM, NOT A DIAGNOSIS **

is punctuated by a normally conducted beat. Dissociation can of course also develop between the atria and an independent ectopic ventricular rhythm (fig. 179); and occasionally even between two A-V junctional pacemakers, the one controlling the atria and the other the ventricles.

When the two independent pacemakers have nearly identical rates, the term **isorhythmic dissociation** is applicable (8) (fig. 178 A).

But A-V dissociation is nö more a complete diagnosis than is jaundice. Like jaundice it may be the striking feature that catches the eye, but it is always *secondary* to some primary disturbance; and its significance depends upon that of the primary disturbance. In figure 178, the dissociation is just as real in both examples, but in A it is the result of a normal mechanism, sinus bradycardia in an athlete; whereas in B the dissociation is abnormal because it results from enhanced A-V nodal automaticity.

A-V dissociation may be caused by factors which depress the S-A node, such as vagotonia or digitalis; or by abnormal conditions that make the A-V node more excitable, such as rheumatic fever, acute infections and digitalis. It not uncommonly complicates the course of coronary disease. It is important to stress, however, that it may be seen in perfectly normal hearts when physiological sinus bradycardia leads to A-V nodal escape.

This brief discussion of A-V dissociation has oversimplified the subject, but a more detailed discussion is beyond the intended scope of this book. The whole subject has been fully reviewed (2, 3, 6, 7) and readers who wish to pursue its ramifications and entanglements further are referred to these articles.

REFERENCES

1. Katz, L. N., and Pick, A.: *Clinical Electrocardiography. The Arrhythmias.* Lea and Febiger, Philadelphia, 1956.
2. Marriott, H. J. L., et al.: A-V dissociation: a re-appraisal. Am. J. Cardiol. 1958: **2**, 586.
3. Menendez, M. M., and Marriott, H. J. L.: A-V dissociation revisited. Progr. Cardiovasc. Dis. 1966: **8**, 522.
4. Pick, A.: Aberrant ventricular conduction of escaped beats. Preferential and accessory pathways in the A-V junction. Circulation 1956: **13**, 702.
5. Pick, A., and Dominguez, P.: Nonparoxysmal A-V nodal tachycardia. Circulation 1957: **16**, 1022.
6. Pick, A.: A-V dissociation. A proposal for a comprehensive classification and consistent terminology. Am. Heart J. 1963: **66**, 147.
7. Schott, A.: Atrioventricular dissociation with and without interference. Progr. Cardiovasc. Dis. 1959: **2**, 444.
8. Schubart, A. F., et al.: Isorhythmic dissociation: atrioventricular dissociation with synchronization. Am. J. Med. 1958: **24**, 209.

Review Tracings

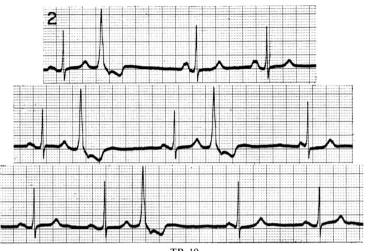

TR-19

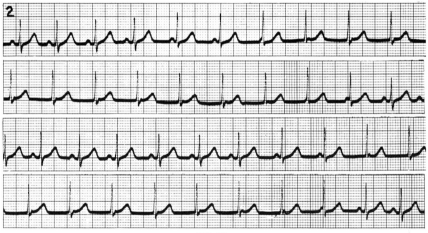

TR-20

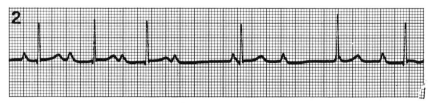

TR-21

For interpretations, see pages 314–17

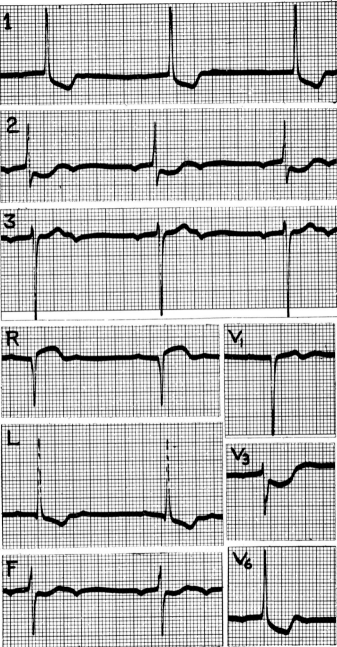

TR-22

For interpretation, see pages 314–17

17

Artificial Pacemakers

The introduction of artificial pacemakers has opened a new chapter in arrhythmias, both by producing their own new crop and by shedding new light on long recognized mechanisms (2). Pacemaker "blips" have become familiar artifacts in the clinical tracing, and figures 180–185 illustrate various patterns of effective and ineffective pacemaker activity.

There are four types of artificial pacemakers (1):

1) Fixed rate—recognized in the electrocardiogram by the fact that pacemaker "blips" occur with relentless regularity, their rhythm unaffected by the intervention of naturally occurring beats (fig. 180).

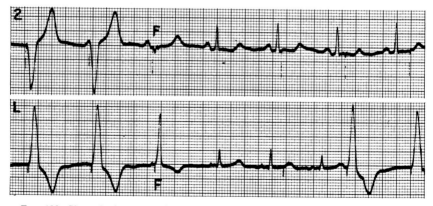

Fig. 180. Sinus rhythm competing with a fixed rate **artificial pacemaker** with resulting fusion beats (F). Note that regular rhythm of pacemaker blips is not disturbed by the natural beats.

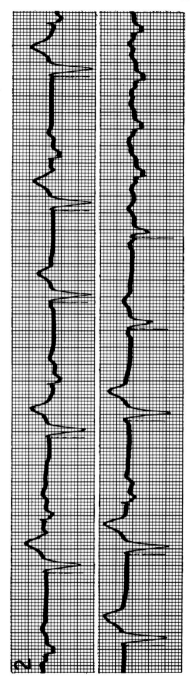

FIG. 181. **Demand pacemaker.** Note that when a natural beat occurs, the pacemaker shuts off. The sinus beats are conducted with intraventricular block and the 5th and 6th beats in the bottom strip are fusion beats. In the top strip, the 1st and 4th paced beats are followed by retrograde P waves which in turn are followed by probable reciprocal beats.

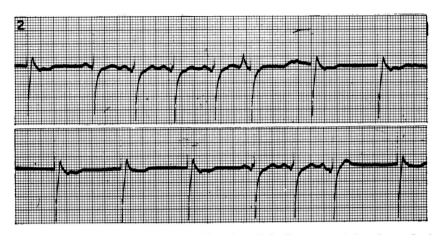

FIG. 182. **Atrial-triggered pacemaker.** Note that all the P waves are followed, at a fixed interval, by a pacemaker "blip." When no P waves appear in time to trigger the pacemaker, the pacemaker functions like a fixed-rate pacemaker at a pre-set rate.

2) Demand (ventricular-inhibited)—recognized by the fact that, when a natural beat occurs, the regular rhythm of the pacemaker blips is interrupted (fig. 181); then, after a predetermined "escape" interval, the pacemaker fires again unless another natural beat anticipates it.

3) Atrial-triggered—recognized by the fact that the blips always follow a P wave at a fixed interval (fig. 182).

4) Ventricular-triggered—this seldom seen pacemaker is recognized by the fact that the blip is in, not immediately before, the QRS complex of natural beats.

Notes: a) If there are no natural beats (fig. 183), you cannot distinguish between a fixed rate and demand pacemaker; because the demand pacemaker, if it is not interrupted by natural beats, will continue to fire regularly. b) The demand pacemaker operates exactly like a ventricular escape rhythm, whereas the fixed rate pacemaker functions like ventricular parasystole. Both are therefore potent manufacturers of fusion beats. c) Both atrial-triggered and ventricular-triggered pacemakers become demand pacemakers when there are no natural complexes to trigger them.

A normally functioning transvenous pacemaker produced figure 183. Like other electrocardiographic manifestations of electrical activity, the pacemaker spike has magnitude and direction and, though easily seen in most leads, may be inconspicuous or quite invisible in others (fig. 185).

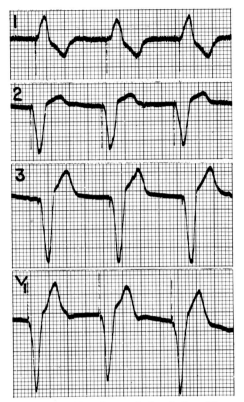

FIG. 183. Ectopic ventricular rhythm driven by **artificial pacemaker**—note pacemaker "blip" immediately preceding each QRS. Since the QRS shows marked left axis deviation, the pacemaker is situated in the right ventricle (transvenous pacemaker).

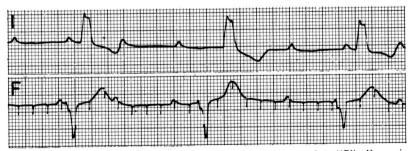

FIG. 184. Complete A-V block with ineffective **runaway pacemaker.** "Blips" are visible at rate 350 in aVF; note that there is no sign of pacemaker activity in lead 1.

When an artificial pacemaker is only partially effective, or when A-V conduction reappears, the resulting competition may lead to fusion beats and bizarre rhythms (fig. 180). A malfunctioning pacemaker may go berserk and fire at several hundred times per minute (fig. 184), sometimes driving the ventricles in a wild tachycardia.

Like all other ectopic ventricular rhythms, paced rhythms may be associated with retrograde conduction to the atria (figs. 181 and 185).

When the atria are paced, as may be undertaken in the absence of A-V block, the pacemaker blip is immediately followed by a P wave instead of a ventricular complex (fig. 186).

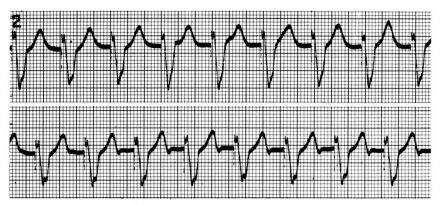

FIG. 185. **Artificial pacemaker** with dissociated atrial activity in the top strip; in the bottom strip, 1:1 retrograde conduction develops (retrograde P waves produce sharp negative deformity at end of T-wave downstroke).

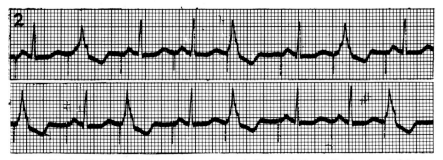

FIG. 186. **Artificial pacemaker** pacing atria: each P wave is immediately preceded by a pacemaker "blip." The paced rhythm is interrupted by frequent ventricular premature beats which happen to coincide with the next expected P waves so that they look like paced ventricular beats.

REFERENCES

1. Castellanos, A., and Lemberg, L.: *Electrophysiology of Pacing and Cardioversion.* Appleton-Century-Crofts, New York, 1969.
2. Katz, A. M., and Pick, A.: The transseptal conduction time in the human heart. Circulation 1963: **27,** 1061.

Review Tracings

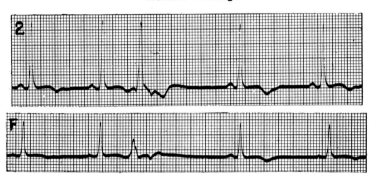

TR-23

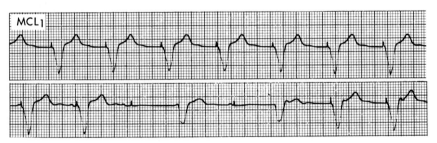

TR-24

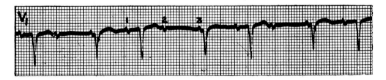

TR-25

For interpretations, see pages 314–17

18

Myocardial Infarction

EXPERIMENTAL CONSIDERATIONS

If a branch of a dog's coronary is tied and an electrode is placed on an area of myocardium supplied by the occluded vessel, the T waves in the derived tracing soon become inverted. If the ligature is then re-moved and the flow of blood to the muscle re-established, the inverted T waves soon return to normal. The T-wave inversion is therefore clearly the result of simple ischemia. Inverted T waves form the basis of the **pattern of ischemia** in the clinical tracing.

If when T inversion occurs the ligature is allowed to remain in place, a dramatic change in the pattern shortly develops: within a minute or two the ST segment becomes strikingly elevated, dragging up with it and obliterating the inverted T wave. If at this stage the tie is removed, the tracing, gradually passing back through the inverted T stage, again reverts to normal. ST elevation, representing a stage beyond ischemia but still reversible, is known as the **pattern of injury.**

If when the pattern of injury is fully developed the tie is left in place, a further striking change eventually occurs. The entire QRS complex becomes inverted to produce a QS complex, while the ST segment comes back to the isoelectric line and the T wave once more assumes its nor-mal upright contour. If this pattern is allowed to persist for long before the ligature is removed, it is found to be irreversible—no matter how long you wait, a QS pattern will continue to be recorded from the damaged area. Irreversible structural changes have occurred, and the new pat-tern is called the **pattern of necrosis.**

The reason necrosis produces Q waves is as follows: If a segment of myocardium is knocked out, electromotive forces cease to traverse it. There is thus a loss of forces directed toward the electrode placed over the inert muscle, and this results in a negative deflection (Q wave). By the same token there will be a relative gain in forces directed away from the inert area, and this may be indicated by increase in the size of the positive deflection (R wave) in leads taken from the opposite surface of the heart. This concept is helpful in explaining some of the less classical patterns of infarction encountered, several of which will be discussed later in this chapter.

CLINICAL INFARCTION

The two main types of infarction used to be called anterior and posterior. But because the term "posterior" is anatomically inaccurate, as it was applied to the surface of the heart resting on the diaphragm, it is becoming more common and certainly better practice to use the terms "inferior" or "diaphragmatic" when referring to lesions of this wall.

If you hold a heart in your hand, it is at once obvious that there are no clearcut surfaces or boundaries; any "walls" defined are at best rough approximations. The four walls usually referred to in discussions of infarction are anterior, lateral, inferior and true posterior (to distinguish it from the false posterior of the older terminology).

The three changes observed in the experimental heart—T-wave inversion, ST elevation and the appearance of Q waves—form the basis of infarction patterns as we see them clinically. Around any patch of infarcted muscle there is a less damaged zone which produces the pattern of injury; and outside this an even less affected area which produces the pattern of ischemia. In the experimental heart these zones can be "tapped" individually with small electrodes placed directly on the epicardium (**direct leads**). Clinically the nearest one can get is several centimeters from the myocardium on the outside of the chest (**semi-direct leads**). A natural result of this is that the precordial pattern is usually a composite picture combining the patterns of ischemia, injury and necrosis all in one QRST sequence—the relatively distant electrode is influenced by all three zones instead of only one.

The first step, then, in diagnosing infarction from the electrocardiogram is to know what changes to look for. Those changes are 1) the **fresh appearance of Q waves or the increased prominence of pre-existing ones,** 2) **ST segment elevations** and 3) **T-wave inversions.** Only Q-wave changes are diagnostic of infarction (necrosis), but changes in the ST segments and T waves may be suspicious and provide strong presumptive evidence. The Q, ST and T changes all have special characteristics:

The Q wave is often wide as well as deep; any Q measuring 0.03 sec. or more in width is highly suspicious of infarction. The deviated ST segments typically show an upward convexity. The fully developed T waves are pointed and consist of two symmetrical limbs, well likened to an arrowhead. These three changes are summarized in figure 187. Note that these changes are registered in **leads that face the area of damage**, and it is convenient to refer to them collectively as "indicative" changes. Opposite, or "reciprocal," changes (i.e., no Q wave with perhaps some increase in height of R wave, depressed ST segments and tall upright T waves) meanwhile appear in leads facing the diametrically opposed surface of the heart. Fortified with a little imagination and with a glance at

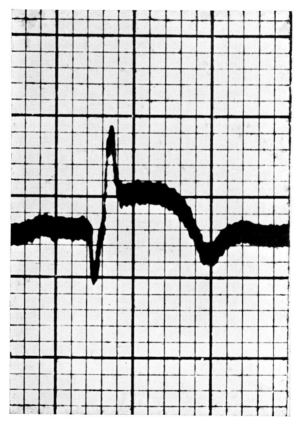

FIG. 187. **Acute myocardial infarction.** The three indicative changes—Q wave, ST elevation and T inversion.

figure 188, it is relatively simple to decide what changes will occur in which leads when various surfaces of the heart are involved. Leads whose positive poles face the inferior surface (2, 3 and aVF) are most important in the diagnosis of **inferior** infarction. Reciprocal changes are usually seen in leads 1, aVL and some of the precordial leads. In **anterior** infarction indicative changes occur in precordial leads and in leads 1 and aVL, while reciprocal changes develop in leads 2, 3 and aVF. In **lateral** wall infarction leads 1, aVL and V_5 and V_6 are most likely to show indicative changes, and reciprocal changes may sometimes develop in leads taken farthest to the right (V_1, V_{3R}, etc.). None of the routine 12 leads faces the **true posterior** surface of the heart, and so infarction of this wall must be inferred from reciprocal changes occurring in anterior leads, especially V_1 and V_2.

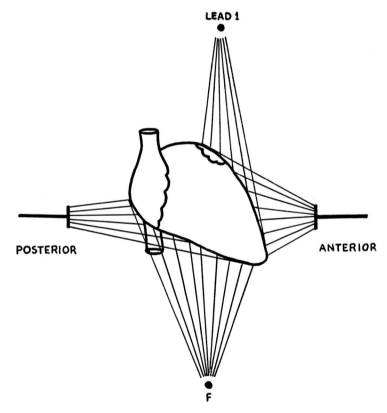

LEAD 1

POSTERIOR

ANTERIOR

F

FIG. 188. Illustrating how the anterior chest leads and lead 1 both face the same "anterior" (really anterosuperior) surface of the heart, while the posterior chest leads and the positive pole (F) of leads 2, 3 and aVF face the inferior (diaphragmatic) surface.

The limb lead patterns associated with the two main types of infarction, anterior and inferior, are perhaps worth summarizing separately. Anterior infarction produces indicative changes in lead 1 and for this reason is sometimes called Q_1T_1 type infarction. Inferior infarction produces indicative changes in lead 3 and is therefore called Q_3T_3 type infarction. In anterior infarction indicative changes are also seen in aVL and reciprocal changes appear in 2, 3 and aVF. In inferior infarction indicative changes are also found in 2, 3 and aVF, while reciprocal changes develop in 1 and aVL. These changes are summarized in figure 189. Remember, however, that the characteristic changes of infarction may appear *only* in the precordial leads, the limb leads remaining normal or near normal.

Evaluation of Q_3

As a prominent Q wave in lead 3 is one of the hallmarks of inferior infarction but is also sometimes a normal finding, its evaluation is often difficult (9). It is more likely to be abnormal if it is wide (more than 0.03 sec.), if it is associated with Q waves also in 2 and aVF, and if it is followed by a slurred upstroke into the R wave.

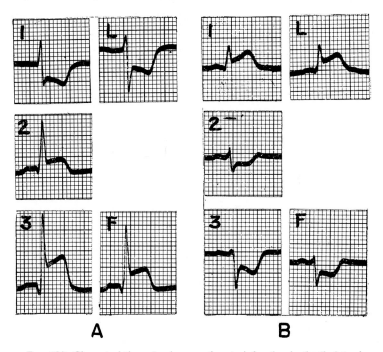

A   **B**

FIG. 189. Characteristic early changes of acute infarction in the limb leads. A. Inferior infarction. B. Anterior infarction.

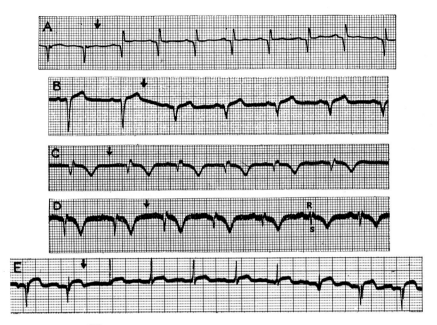

FIG. 190. Effect of deep inspiration on Q_3 in patients with inferior infarction. Inspiration began at the arrow in each strip. Note that there is relatively
little effect on the negative wave in A, B, C and D. In D the Q wave is replaced
by a small initial R wave, but an appreciable negative (S) wave persists. In E,
however, the pathological Q wave is entirely drawn up.

A simple test is sometimes helpful: deep inspiration will usually cause an
innocuous (positional) Q_3 to disappear or materially decrease; whereas the
Q_3 of infarction is relatively unaffected by this simple maneuver (4) (fig.
190 A).

At times, but by no means invariably, it is helpful to refer the decision
to the aV leads (37), for lead 3, connecting left arm and left leg, represents
the difference between aVF and aVL (3 = aVF − aVL). If the initial deflection of the QRS in aVF is less positive (or more negative) than the
corresponding deflection in aVL, there will be an initial negative (Q) wave

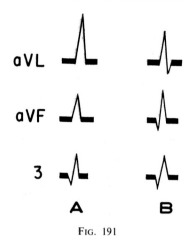

FIG. 191

in 3. And so if there is no Q wave in either aVL or aVF but the R wave
in aVF is not so tall as the R in aVL (fig. 191A), there will be a Q wave
in 3. This will clearly not be a pathological Q wave, as it results simply
from difference in the height of normal R waves. In such a situation the
aV leads give an immediate favorable answer. If on the other hand there
is a Q wave in aVF (fig 191 B), one has merely transferred the burden of
proof to aVF and it then has to be decided whether the Q there is of abnormal significance or not.

Salient Features of Acute Myocardial Infarction

	Anterior	Inferior
1. Indicative changes (Q, ST elevation, T inversion) in leads:	1, aVL, anterior chest	2, 3, aVF, posterior chest
2. Reciprocal changes in leads:	2, 3, aVF, posterior chest	1, aVL, anterior chest
3. Progressive changes in pattern from day to day		

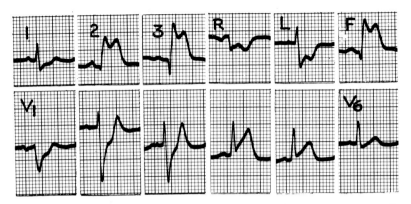

Fig. 192. Acute **infero-apical** myocardial infarction. Note ST elevation in 2, 3, aVF, V_4 and V_5 with reciprocal depression in other leads. Q waves are developing in 2, 3 and aVF.

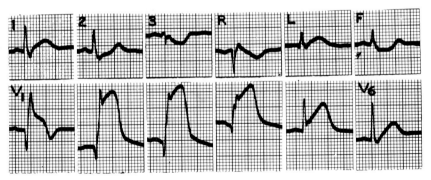

Fig. 193. **Acute anterior myocardial infarction.** Note ST elevation in V_{1-5}, and loss of the normal upward concavity of the ST segment in 1, aVL and V_6, with reciprocal changes in 2, 3 and aVF. Q waves have developed in the right chest leads, and the pattern of RBBB has appeared, indicating septal involvement.

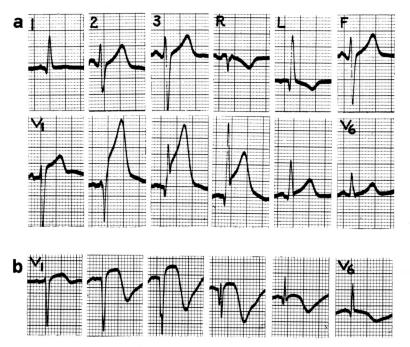

Fig. 194. **Acute extensive anterior myocardial infarction.** In **a**, note probable left anterior hemiblock in the limb leads with high ST take-off and tall T waves in precordial leads; in **b**, 2 days later, "coving" of ST segments with deep inversion of T and U waves, while simultaneously R waves have dwindled in V_{1-2}, a QS complex has appeared in V_3, and Q waves have developed or deepened in V_{4-6}.

Further observations

Some important general points:

1. *Time relationships* are important. Rarely, no changes develop in the tracing for several days or even for two or three weeks. Usually, however, they begin to make their appearance within the first few hours. ST-segment changes appear early and progress. At this stage the T waves, later to become inverted, actually become taller and appear as an upward extension of the rising ST segments (25) (figs. 194 and 195). This early tall T wave may be mistaken for the later tall T wave of reciprocal leads, and an early anterior infarction may thus be wrongly labelled as inferior. Some-

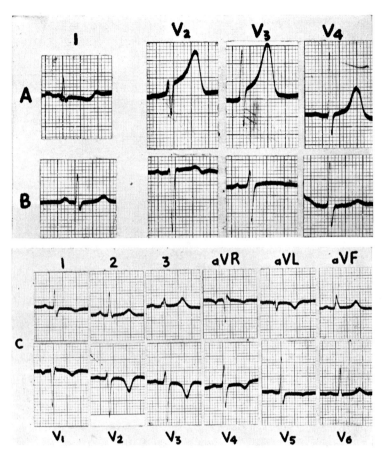

Fig. 195. A. **Acute anteroseptal myocardial infarction.** Note the tall T waves in V_{2-4}, where they will later be deeply inverted. B. Taken just a few hours later; note striking changes in T waves; tracing is now remarkably normal. C. Taken 6 days later; shows fully developed pattern of anteroseptal infarction. Note that no pathological Q waves have developed, but the infarction can be diagnosed with certainty from the striking evolution in the ST-T pattern.

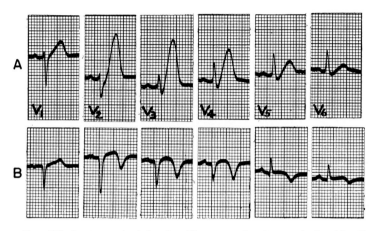

FIG. 196. Acute **anterior infarction.** Note unusual early stage in A, with tall T waves and *depressed* ST take-off. B, taken a few days later, shows typical evolution of anterior infarction.

times this tall T wave is associated with striking depression of the ST segment (30), and then of course the reciprocal pattern of an inferior infarction is even more closely simulated (fig. 196 A). To add to the confusion similar tall T waves are occasionally seen as an early stage of inferior infarction (8); in such cases this may well represent a premonitory stage of diaphragmatic wall ischemia before actual infarction has occurred. Similar but persistent tall T waves are a not uncommon finding in patients with angina (33) (see chapter 19, fig. 212).

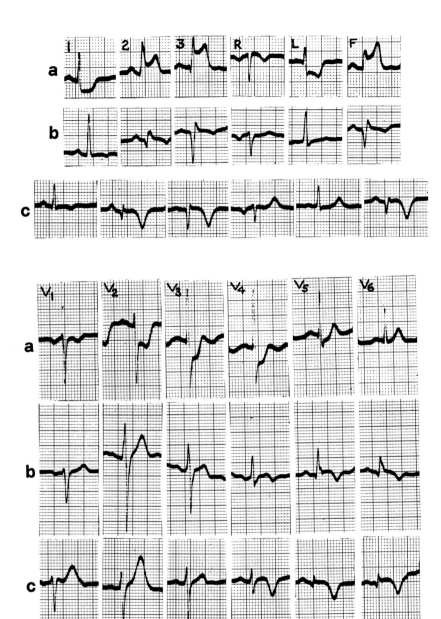

FIG. 197. **Acute inferolateral myocardial infarction.** Tracing a was taken 3 days before b, and b 6 days before c. Note in a indicative changes in 2, 3 and aVF with reciprocal changes in 1, aVL and the chest leads V_{2-5}. Subsequent evolution demonstrates indicative changes in the left chest leads as well, so that the infarction is inferolateral. Note also that the QRS axis shifts from about $+60°$ to $-30°$ (thanks to the development of infarction Q waves, not to left anterior hemiblock) and that the R waves in left chest leads have shrunk away.

Q waves may appear early or may not develop for several days. Whenever the various changes appear they tend to evolve in a fairly typical sequence (fig. 198). In the indicative leads the ST segments rise higher and higher and then begin to return to the baseline, while the T waves develop progressively deeper inversion; finally, after weeks or months, the T waves may become shallower and finally return to normal. Thus ST changes are usually the most transitory; the T changes are more lasting; but the Q

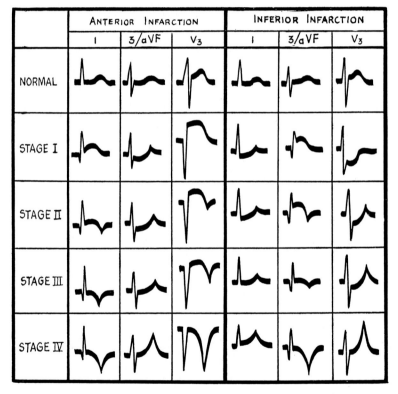

Fig. 198. **Acute myocardial infarction.** Stages of evolution in the patterns of anterior and inferior infarctions.

waves are the most likely to remain as a permanent record of the my-ocardial scar. Even well established Q waves, however, may at times completely disappear. Persistent ST segment elevation (31) (fig. 199) or the presence of an rsR' pattern in V_6 (32) suggest the possibility of ventricular aneurysm.

The model sequence of changes depicted diagrammatically in figure 198 is not invariable, but there is always some "evolution" of the pattern along similar lines, and to diagnose an *acute* infarction such evolution must be in evidence. For there is no means of being certain, in a single tracing, whether the typical changes of infarction are due to an acute process or are the remnants of an old one. ST segment deviations are least likely to represent an old process, but even they may sometimes endure for a long time and rarely are permanent. Progressive changes from day to day are the conclusive evidence of an active, acute process.

2. The electrocardiogram should be considered *confirmatory* of the clinical impression, and should not supersede it. If the patient is suspected clinically of having sustained a myocardial infarct, he should be treated accordingly even if his tracing is completely normal. The looked-for changes may be late to appear or, rarely, they may never appear in the routine leads although the infarction is a clinical certainty. For factors favoring missed diagnoses, see page 246.

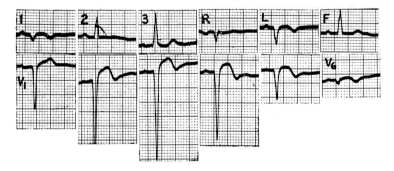

FIG. 199. Old **anterior myocardial infarction** with persistent ST elevation in precordial leads 3 years after the infarction. A ventricular aneurysm was demonstrated.

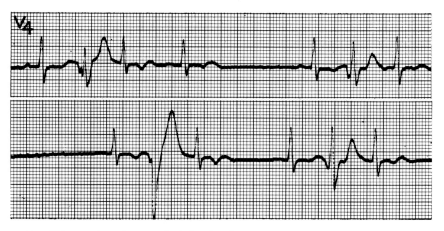

Fig. 200. **Anterior infarction,** the indicative Q waves of which are obvious in the ventricular extrasystoles and absent in the conducted beats. (From a 52-year-old physician who had an anterior infarction two years previously.)

3. The Q waves of infarction may be better revealed in ectopic ventricular beats than in the conducted sinus beats (26, 27) (fig. 200).

4. A T-wave pattern of some importance is the **T_1-lower-than-T_3** pattern. T_1 is often found normally lower than T_3 in vertical hearts. It is also abnormally present in early left ventricular overload, before frank inversion of T_1 has occurred. If both vertical heart and left ventricular overload can be excluded such a pattern is extremely suspicious of an anterior infarction, either old or recent (29).

5. Apart from the changes specific for acute infarction, other abnormalities frequently appear. The tracing often shows low voltage and the QT duration is frequently prolonged, reaching its maximum in the second week. Any arrhythmia or block may develop, and continuously monitored series indicate that some form of rhythm disturbance occurs in 75 to 95 per cent of all patients. In order of frequency, the commonest to develop are ventricular premature beats, supraventricular premature beats, atrial fibrillation, ventricular tachycardia, accelerated idioventricular rhythms and supraventricular tachycardia. A-V block develops much more often in inferior than in anterior infarction.

Complex patterns

Frequently the pattern observed is not so "pure" as the ones so far described. If the anterior and inferior walls of the left ventricle are both involved in the process, **antero-inferior infarction,** varying combinations of the changes typical of each may occur (3). Sometimes an inferior infarction develops in a heart that has suffered a previous anterior infarction, or vice versa; in such circumstances the current infarction, producing changes opposite (or reciprocal) to the changes of the previous infarction, may tend to "normalize" the tracing so that it looks "better" than it did before the second occlusion.

Bundle-branch block, producing as it does bizarre QRS, ST and T changes of its own, may completely mask the changes of a superimposed infarction. One of the most difficult diagnoses to make is that of infarction in the presence of left bundle-branch block (11, 12). If a previous tracing is available showing the uncomplicated block pattern, then the appearance of fresh Q waves (especially over the left ventricle, where they are not found in uncomplicated left bundle-branch block) is good evidence of acute infarction. Q waves in 1, aVL or V_6 in the presence of left bundle-branch block (fig. 205) are strongly suspicious of anteroseptal infarction (15). A decrease in amplitude of R waves over the left ventricle (14), or a change in the elevation or shape of ST segments or T waves, may provide a suspicious clue to acute infarction, but certainty can only be expressed if definite evolution in a pattern suspicious of infarction is noted from day to day.

Right bundle-branch block is less likely to cause confusion (13). Both anterior and inferior infarction patterns can be seen superimposed on the block pattern (figs. 193, 201 and 204). The block may have preceded the infarction or may have resulted from it; indeed, the presence of bundle-branch block may be considered an integral part of the pattern of **septal infarction** (36).

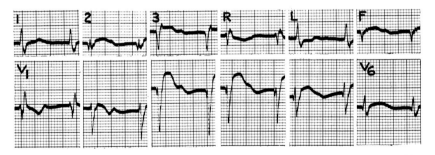

FIG. 201. **Antero-inferior myocardial infarction.** Note that indicative changes are evident in both anterior (V_{2-6}) and inferior (2, 3, and aVF) leads; RBBB has also developed, indicating septal involvement. There is also marked prolongation of the P-R interval to about 0.40 sec. which may well be due to incomplete LBBB.

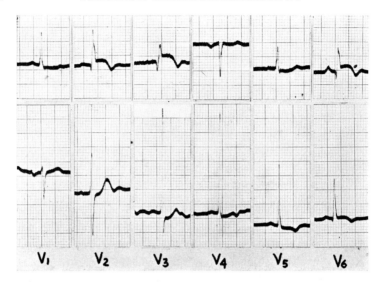

Fig. 202. **Acute inferolateral infarction.** Note indicative changes in 2, 3 and aVF. The ST-T changes in V_6 suggest lateral extension of the infarction.

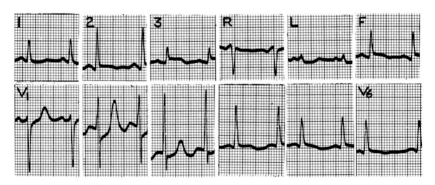

Fig. 203. **Acute inferolateral infarction.** There is ST elevation in 2, 3, aVF and V_{4-6}, with classical reciprocal changes in V_{1-2}.

Localization of infarction

Localization is good academic exercise, but is of relatively little practical value. It is a modest aid to prognosis, for it is generally agreed that the best prognosis is enjoyed by patients with small anteroseptal, lateral or subendocardial infarctions, while septal infarctions producing bundle-branch block and combined anterior and inferior infarctions carry the worst outlook. The most important clinical question, hwever, is "Has an infarction occurred?," not "Where is it?".

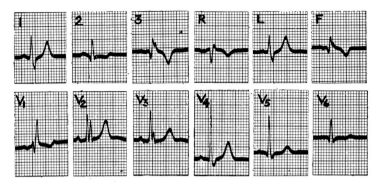

FIG. 204. Acute **inferior infarction** with **right bundle-branch block**. Q and T changes are evident in 2, 3 and aVF, with reciprocal T-wave changes in V_{2-4}.

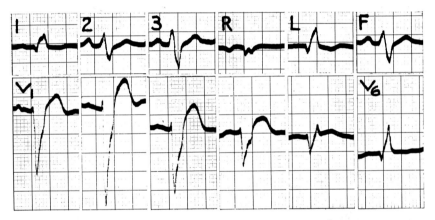

FIG. 205. **Anteroseptal infarction**. The QRS pattern is characteristic of LBBB except that there are unexpected Q waves in 1, aVL and V6.

Localization is mainly based on the previously stated principle that indicative changes (those epitomized in fig. 187, page 228) occur in leads facing the damaged surface of the heart. Thus if indicative changes are seen in all the precordial leads from V_1 to V_6, we diagnose an **extensive anterior** or **anterolateral infarction** (2) (figs. 193, 196 and 199). If such changes occur only in one or more of leads V_1 to V_4, the infarct is labelled **anteroseptal** (1) (fig. 195, page 235). If the limb leads indicate an inferior infarction, but indicative changes are present also in leads V_5 and V_6, we would call it an inferior infarction with lateral extension or an **inferolateral infarct** (7) (figs. 197, 202 and 203). If the only changes seen are in 1 and aVL it would suggest **lateral infarction** (24), and so on.

Subendocardial infarction (16–21) is diagnosed if 1) the clinical picture justifies the diagnosis of infarction, 2) Q waves are absent and 3) several of the limb and precordial leads show ST depression and T wave inversions (fig. 206) that persist.

The subendocardial layer of myocardium is particularly vulnerable because, being close to the ventricular cavity, it is subjected to particularly high pressure during systole and is therefore the earliest zone to "feel the pinch" when coronary adequacy falters.

Infarction without Q waves

Q waves have come to be regarded as the hallowed hallmark of infarction. But there is nothing sacred about Q waves as such. Their importance is that they represent the replacement of electrical forces directed toward the electrode by oppositely directed forces, i.e., replacement of impulses (dipoles) travelling toward the electrode by impulses travelling away from it. This being so, loss of R wave with or without gain in depth of S wave might well carry the same significance as a Q wave. Indeed, in some circumstances this is true. Loss of QRS amplitude over the left ventricle has already been mentioned as a clue to infarction in the presence of left bundle-branch block.

Again, reversal of the normal trend in height of R waves in the first three or four precordial leads may be a helpful sign. In these leads we have seen that the height of the R wave normally increases from right to left. If, however, these R waves dwindle progressively from right to left it is suspicious of anteroseptal infarction. But even complete loss of R waves (i.e., QS complexes) in V_1 through V_4 is not necessarily evidence of anterior infarction and is sometimes seen in left ventricular hypertrophy (see below)

In true posterior or inferoposterior infarction the only changes may be reciprocal ones observed in the anterior chest leads. At times in true posterior or in lateral infarction (21, 23) the sole or primary change may be an increase in the height of R waves over the right precordium (V_{3R}, V_1, V_2). Similarly, an increased width of the R wave to 0.04 sec. or more in V_1 and V_2 may be diagnostic of true posterior infarction (5) (fig. 207).

Another infarction pattern, of which the most striking feature is *left axis deviation*, was described by Grant (34). Its characteristics are 1) an initial wide R wave (0.04 sec. or more) followed by a deep S wave in aVF, and 2) marked left axis deviation of more than $-30°$. A careful study with autopsy correlation showed that many patients with this pattern had infarction of the anterolateral wall. He attributed the axis shift to "peri-infarction block," but subsequent work (28) indicates that this pattern is more

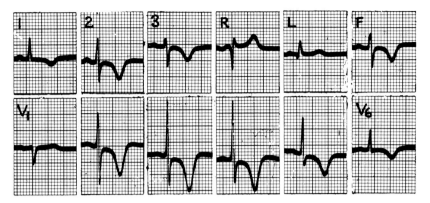

FIG. 206. **Acute subendocardial infarction.** From a patient with the clinical picture of infarction; note widespread ST-T depression in limb and chest leads, but no associated Q waves.

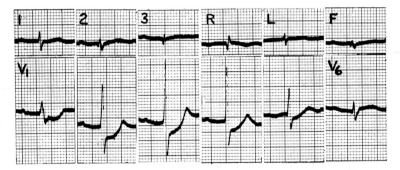

FIG. 207. Probable **acute true posterior infarction.** Note prominent and wide R waves in V_1 and other right precordial leads accompanied by reciprocal ST-T changes in the same leads; these features in anterior leads suggest an acute infarction of the opposite, i.e., posterior, wall.

often found with LVH or diffuse scarring of the left ventricle than with a discrete infarction. Its probable anatomic basis is left anterior hemiblock (see p. 86).

Grant also pointed out that *right axis deviation* may sometimes result from infarction of the diaphragmatic wall (5); the probable explanation for this is left posterior hemiblock.

One of the listed criteria for diagnosing a subendocardial infarction was absence of Q waves. The explanation for this finding is that the impulse travels much faster (several thousand millimeters per second) through the inner third of the myocardium than through the outer two thirds (about

500 mm. per second). In fact it travels so fast that it makes no impression on the depolarization complex (QRS) as recorded by our crude instruments; experimentally and in the human heart the QRS remains unaltered when the inner myocardial layers alone are injured (18, 19).

It is thus clear that Q waves, although they remain the sheet anchor of confident diagnosis, are by no means a sine qua non of all infarction patterns.

Q waves without infarction

Just as the absence of Q waves does not exclude, so their presence does not prove, infarction. One of the commonest errors of over-interpretation is in the reading of anteroseptal infarction from QS complexes in V_1 and V_2—a pattern much more often produced by left ventricular hypertrophy alone. The following conditions can produce pathological Q waves that simulate those of myocardial infarction:
  1. Ventricular hypertrophy, left or right (43, 48)
  2. Diffuse myocardial disease (44, 45, 49)
  3. Localized myocardial replacement
  4. Acute extracardiac catastrophes, e.g., pancreatitis (40), pulmonary embolism, pneumonia (42), etc.
  5. Ventricular pre-excitation (50)
In addition, significant Q waves may occur as a transient manifestation of myocardial ischemia (47); and they are rarely seen in apparently normal youths (41).

Concluding notes on diagnosis

It should be remembered that the accentuating effect of the CF connection on negative deflections (page 5) may profitably be exploited to bring out the pattern of anterior myocardial damage. Abnormal T-wave changes may appear earlier, be more conclusive and persist longer in the CF than the V leads (figs. 208 and 4, page 6).

Finally, let us remind ourselves that the electrocardiogram is not infallible in the diagnosis of infarction. It has been estimated that with 12 routine leads only 80 to 90 per cent of cases are diagnosable. Factors to bear in mind as probable causes of missed diagnoses are:
  1. Failure to take serial tracings
  2. Failure to take additional exploratory chest leads in doubtful cases
  3. Presence of bundle-branch block
  4. Digitalis action tending to neutralize ST elevations
  5. Simultaneous infarcts neutralizing each other's patterns

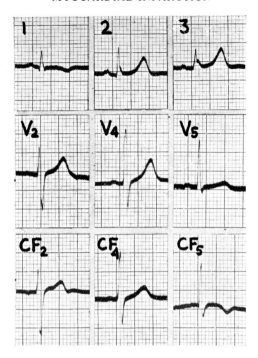

Fig. 208. Comparison of V and CF leads in an
early **anterior infarction;** note that while the V leads
are entirely normal, CF₅ shows an obviously abnormal T wave.

ATRIAL INFARCTION

Infarction of the atrium must be suspected when, in the presence of ventricular infarction, an atrial arrhythmia develops. Other criteria include
elevation of the P-R segment in left chest leads with reciprocal depression
in right chest leads; elevation of the P-R segment in lead 1 with reciprocal
depression in lead 3; widespread depression of the P-R segment in the
presence of an atrial arrhythmia; abnormal P-wave contour (51).

REFERENCES

ANTERIOR INFARCTION

1. Myers, G. B., Klein, H. A., and Stofer, B. E.: Correlation of electrocardiographic and
   pathologic findings in anteroseptal infarction. Am. Heart J. 1948: **36,** 535.
2. Myers, G. B., Klein, H. A., and Hiratzka, T.: Correlation of electrocardiographic and
   pathologic findings in large anterolateral infarcts. Am. Heart J. 1948: **36,** 838.
3. Myers, G. B., Klein, H. A., and Hiratzka, T.: Correlation of electrocardiographic and
   pathologic findings in anteroposterior infarction. Am. Heart J. 1949: **37,** 205.

INFERIOR (FORMERLY "POSTERIOR") INFARCTION

4. Evans, W.: The effect of deep inbreathing on lead III of the electrocardiogram. Brit. Heart J. 1951: **13**, 457.
5. Grant, R. P., and Murray, R. H.: QRS complex deformity of myocardial infarction in the human subject, Am. J. Med. 1954: **17**, 587.
6. Myers, G. B., Klein, H. A., and Hiratzka, T.: Correlation of electrocardiographic and pathologic findings in posterior infarction. Am. Heart J. 1949: **38**, 547.
7. Myers, G. B., Klein, H. A., and Hiratzka, T.: Correlation of electrocardiographic and pathologic findings in posterolateral infarction. Am. Heart. J. 1949: **38**, 837.
8. Wachtel, F. W., and Teich, E. M.: Tall precordial T waves as the earliest sign of diaphragmatic wall infarction. Am. Heart J. 1956: **51**, 91.
9. Weisbart, M. H., and Simonson, E.: The diagnostic accuracy of Q_3 and related electrocardiographic items for the detection of patients with posterior wall myocardial infarction. Am. Heart J. 1955: **50**, 62.
10. Yu, P. N. G., and Blake, T. M.: The significance of QaVF in the diagnosis of posterior infarction. Am. Heart J. 1950: **40**, 545.

INFARCTION COMPLICATED BY BBB

11. Besoain-Santander, M., and Gomez-Ebensperguer, G.: Electrocardiographic diagnosis of myocardial infarction in cases of complete left bundle branch block. Am. Heart J. 1960: **60**, 886.
12. Dressler, W., Roesler, H., and Schwager, A.: The electrocardiographic signs of myocardial infarction in the presence of bundle branch block. I. Myocardial infarction with left bundle branch block. Am. Heart J. 1950: **39**, 217.
13. Dressler, W., Roesler, H., and Schwager, A.: The electrocardiographic signs of myocardial infarction in the presence of bundle branch block. II. Myocardial infarction with right bundle branch block. Am. Heart J. 1950: **39**, 544.
14. Kennamer, R., and Prinzmetal, M.: Myocardial infarction complicated by left bundle branch block. Am. Heart J. 1956: **51**, 78.
15. Rhoads, D. V., et al.: The electrocardiogram in the presence of myocardial infarction and intraventricular block of the left bundle-branch block type. Am. Heart J. 1961: **62**, 78.

SUBENDOCARDIAL INFARCTION

16. Cook, R. W., et al.: Electrocardiographic changes in acute subendocardial infarction. I. Large subendocardial and nontransmural infarcts. Circulation 1958: **18**, 603. II. Small subendocardial infarcts. Ibid.: 613.
17. Levine, H. D., and Ford, R. V.: Subendocardial infarction: report of six cases and critical survey of the literature. Circulation 1950: **1**, 246.
18. Massumi, R. A., et al.: Studies on the mechanism of ventricular activity. XVI. Activation of the human ventricle. Am. J. Med. 1955: **19**, 832.
19. Prinzmetal, M., et al.: Studies on the mechanism of ventricular activity. VI. The depolarization complex in pure subendocardial infarction; role of the subendocardial region in the normal electrocardiogram. Am. J. Med. 1954: **16**, 469.
20. Pruitt, R. D., Klakeg, C. H., and Chapin, L. E.: Certain clinical states and pathologic changes associated with deeply inverted T waves in the precordial electrocardiogram. Circulation 1955: **11**: 517.
21. Yu, P. N. G., and Stewart, J. M.: Subendocardial myocardial infarction with special reference to the electrocardiographic changes. Am. Heart J. 1950: **39**, 862.

LATERAL INFARCTION

22. Dunn, W. J., Edwards, J. E., and Pruitt, R. D.: The electrocardiogram in infarction of the lateral wall of the left ventricle: a clinicopathologic study. Circulation 1956: **14**, 540.
23. Levy, L., et al.: Prominent R wave and shallow S wave in lead V_1 as a result of lateral myocardial infarction. Am. Heart J. 1950: **40**, 447.
24. Myers, G. B., Klein, H. A., and Stofer, B. E.: Correlation of electrocardiographic and pathologic findings in lateral infarction. 1949: **37**, 374.

MISCELLANEOUS

25. Bayley, R. H., LaDue, J. S., and York, D. J.: Electrocardiographic changes (local ventricular ischemia and injury) produced in the dog by temporary occlusion of a coronary artery, showing a new stage in the evolution of a myocardial infarction. Am. Heart J. 1944: **27**, 164.
26. Benchimol, A., et al.: The ventricular premature contraction. Its place in the diagnosis of ischemic heart disease. Am. Heart J. 1963: **65**, 334.
27. Bisteni, A., et al.: Ventricular premature beats in the diagnosis of myocardial infarction. Brit. Heart J. 1961: **23**, 521.
28. Castle, C. H., and Keane, W. M.: Electrocardiographic "peri-infarction block." A clinical and pathologic correlation. Circulation 1965: **31**, 403.
29. Dressler, W., and Roesler, H.: The diagnostic value of the pattern T_1 lower than T_3 ($T_1 < T_3$) compared with the information yielded by multiple chest leads in myocardial infarction. Am. Heart J. 1948: **36**, 115.
30. Dressler, W., and Roesler, H.: High T waves in the earliest stage of myocardial infarction. Am. Heart J. 1947: **34**, 627.
31. East, T., and Oram, S.: The cardiogram in ventricular aneurysm following cardiac infarction. Brit. Heart J. 1952: **14**, 125.
32. El-Sherif, N.: The rsR′ pattern in left surface leads in ventricular aneurysm. Brit. Heart J. 1970: **32**, 440.
33. Freundlich, J.: The diagnostic significance of tall upright T waves in the chest leads. Am. Heart J. 1956: **52**, 749.
34. Grant, R. P.: Left axis deviation. An electrocardiographic-pathologic correlation study. Circulation 1956: **14**, 233.
35. Grant, R. P.: Peri-infarction block. Progr. Cardiovasc. Dis. 1959: **2**, 237.
36. Osher, H. L., and Wolff, L.: The diagnosis of infarction of the interventricular septum. Am. Heart J. 1953: **45**, 429.
37. Sokolow, M.: The clinical value of the unipolar extremity (aV) leads. Ann. Int. Med. 1951: **34**, 921.
38. Surawicz, B., et al.: QS- and QR-pattern in leads V_3 and V_4 in absence of myocardial infarction: electrocardiographic and vectorcardiographic study. Circulation 1956: **12**, 391.

Q WAVES WITHOUT INFARCTION

39. Class, R. N., et al.: Diphtheritic myocarditis simulating myocardial infarction. Am. J. Cardiol. 1965: **16**, 580.
40. Fulton, M. C., and Marriott, H. J. L.: Acute pancreatitis simulating myocardial infarction in the electrocardiogram. Ann. Int. Med. 1963: **59**, 730.

41. Likoff, W., et al.: Myocardial infarction patterns in young subjects with normal coronary arteriograms. Circulation 1962: **26,** 373.

42. Mamlin, J. J., et al.: Electrocardiographic pattern of massive myocardial infarction without pathologic confirmation. Circulation 1964: **30,** 539.

43. Myers, G. B.: QRS-T patterns in multiple precordial leads that may be mistaken for myocardial infarction. Circulation 1950: **1,** 844 and 860.

44. Oram, S., and Stokes, W.: The heart in scleroderma. Brit. Heart J. 1961: **23,** 243.

45. Perez-Trevino, C., et al.: Glycogen storage disease of the heart. Am. J. Cardiol. 1965: **16,** 137.

46. Pruitt, R. D., et al.: Simulation of electrocardiogram of apicolateral myocardial infarction by myocardial destructive lesions of obscure etiology (myocardiopathy). Circulation 1962: **25,** 506.

47. Rubin, I. L., et al.: Transient abnormal Q waves during coronary insufficiency. Am. Heart J. 1966: **71,** 254.

48. Surawicz, B., et al.: QS- and QR-patterns in leads V_3 and V_4 in absence of myocardial infarction: electrocardiographic and vectorcardiographic study. Circulation 1955: **12,** 391.

49. Tavel, M. E., and Fisch, C.: Abnormal Q waves simulating myocardial infarction in diffuse myocardial diseases. Am. Heart J. 1964: **68,** 534.

50. Wasserburger, R. H., et al.: Noninfarctional $QS_{2, 3, aVF}$ complexes as seen in the Wolff-Parkinson-White syndrome and left bundle branch block. Am. Heart J. 1962: **64,** 617.

ATRIAL INFARCTION

51. Liu, C. K.: Atrial infarction of the heart. Circulation 1961: **23,** 331.

Review Tracings

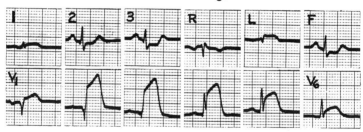

TR-26

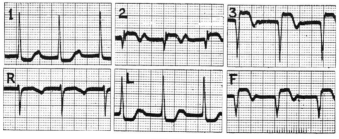

TR-27

For interpretations, see pages 314–17

Review Tracing

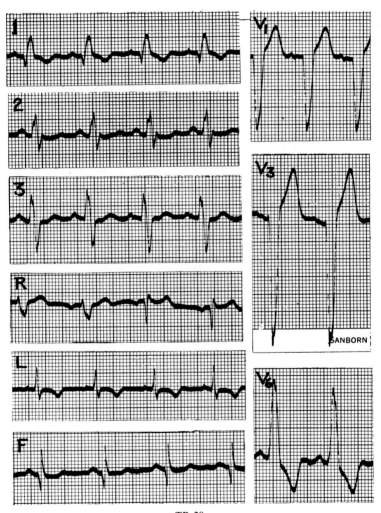

TR-28
For interpretations, see pages 314–17

Review Tracing

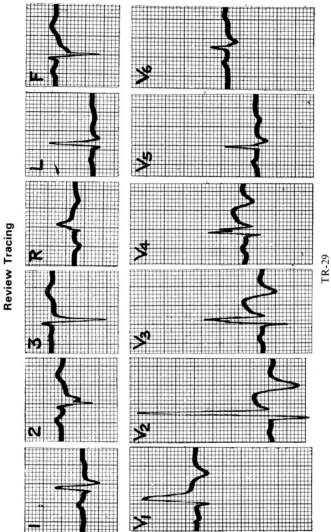

TR-29

For interpretation, see pages 314–17

Review Tracing

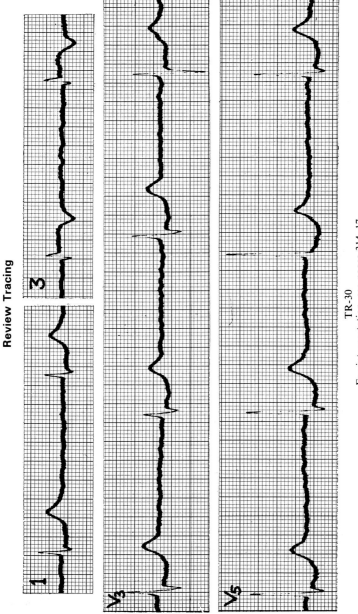

TR-30

For interpretation, see pages 314–17

19

Coronary Insufficiency and Related Matters

Coronary insufficiency may be suspected when T waves are flattened or inverted in many leads, with or without accompanying ST depression (figs. 209 and 210). But a number of other conditions cause ST-T changes which may readily be confused with those of coronary disease. These will be dealt with later in this chapter.

An ST-T pattern particularly suggestive of coronary insufficiency is a horizontal ST segment (also known as "plane" depression (5)) making a sharp angle with the proximal shoulder of the still upright T wave (figs. 209 and 210). Normally the ST segment and T wave should merge smoothly and imperceptibly.

At times the most striking or only evidence of coronary insufficiency is inverted U waves (fig. 211). At other times pathologically tall precordial T

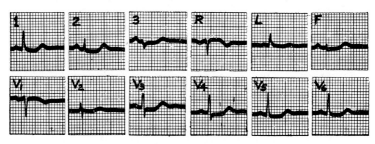

FIG. 209. **Coronary insufficiency.** Note horizontally depressed ST segments in many leads.

254

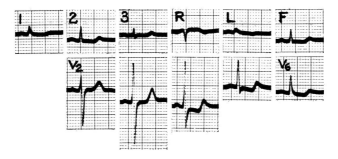

FIG. 210. **Coronary insufficiency.** ST depression in many leads with sharp-angled ST-T junctions.

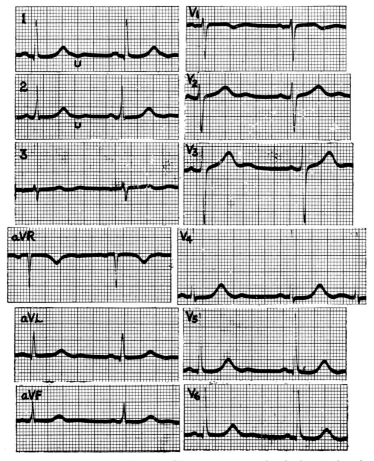

FIG. 211. **Coronary insufficiency.** ST segments are rather horizontal, but the striking abnormality is U-wave inversion, most pronounced in leads 1 and 2.

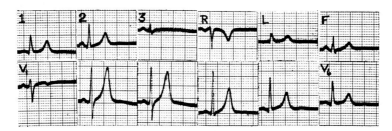

FIG. 212. **Coronary insufficiency.** Abnormally tall precordial T waves are the only electrocardiographic sign of myocardial ischemia in a patient with typical angina.

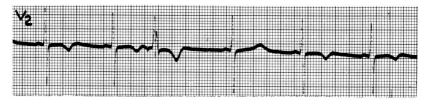

FIG. 213. **Post-extrasystolic T-wave** change. After two sinus beats comes a supraventricular premature beat with ventricular aberration. The sinus beat *following* the extrasystole shows a complete change in polarity of the T wave with prolongation of the Q-T interval.

waves are the sole manifestation of myocardial ischemia (fig. 212).

Another helpful sign of coronary insufficiency is a post-extrasystolic T-wave change (14, 16). The T wave of the sinus beat following the premature beat changes form and often polarity; sometimes this is accompanied by abnormal lengthening of the Q-T interval (fig. 213). Levine has called this the "poor man's exercise test" since the change is included in the initial tracing and so obviates the need and expense of a subsequent exercise test. Useful as this change may be in drawing attention to the possibility of myocardial disease, there is little doubt that it is also sometimes seen in normal hearts (6).

Another minor sign which may direct attention to the presence of coronary disease is the TV$_1$-taller-than-TV$_6$ pattern. In most normal hearts the T wave in V$_6$ is taller than the T wave in V$_1$, which indeed is often inverted. If TV$_1$ is not only upright but taller than TV$_6$, it suggests an abnormality of the left ventricular myocardium and is seen in left ventricular overloading as well as coronary disease (18).

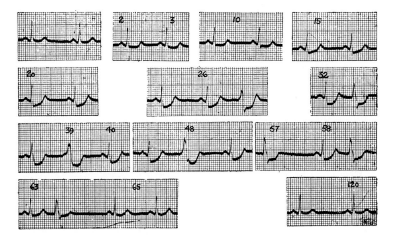

FIG. 214. **Coronary insufficiency.** Lead 2 taken during an attack of chest pain which lasted less than a minute. Top left corner strip taken shortly before pain began spontaneously; figures on subsequent strips represent number of seconds after onset of pain. Notice marked progressive ST-T depression and appearance of frequent ectopic ventricular beats. At the end of 2 min. pattern has returned to normal.

In some cases of coronary insufficiency, abnormalities in the electrocardiogram like those described above occur only *during* an attack of pain (fig. 214). In the "variant form" of angina (19), paradoxical ST *elevation* develops. In other patients, the inadequacy of the coronary circulation can be demonstrated only after exercise (13, 22, 23) or after a period of anoxia, and this is the basis for the various exercise and anoxia tests. The electrocardiogram being normal or borderline while the patient is at rest, he is subjected to exercise or to an atmosphere deficient in oxygen, and tracings are again taken. The appearance of ST depression of 1 mm. or so, with or without flattened or inverted T waves, or any of the other abnormal patterns described above, indicates coronary insufficiency (fig. 215). ST-T *elevation* after exercise probably denotes severe ischemia verging on infarction (7).

Formulas have been devised for the recognition of ischemic heart disease after exercise, but the best criterion remains the ST-T configuration. The rather popular QX/QT ratio (12) is probably unreliable (21). Although post-exercise changes are highly diagnostic of ischemic disease in the clinical suspect, they are not specific, since patterns indistinguishable from those typical of ischemia develop after exercise in other forms of heart disease (9). It is therefore better to say that the typical changes indicate myocardial *disease*, often but not necessarily ischemic.

One must be cautious in interpreting the post-exercise tracing of hypertensive patients receiving thiazides. These drugs may reduce the patient's potassium stores without altering the electrocardiogram; in such a situation, exercise may bring to light the latent pattern of hypokalemia (8), whose ST depression may be mistaken for myocardial ischemia.

The most informative single lead is V_5; but a block of six leads recorded in the following order—V_6, V_5, V_4, V_3, aVF, 2—gives best results (2). The most important tracing is the one taken *immediately* after exercise; later tracings rarely show significant changes in the absence of changes in the immediate tracing (3). Whether monitoring the tracing *during* exercise by radioelectrocardiography (1) will prove diagnostically superior remains to be seen. ST-T changes may result solely from the upright posture and these must not be mistaken for displacements indicating ischemia (10). The "graded" exercise test aims at standardizing the load on the coronary circulation (which, after all, is what is being tested) rather than that on the skeletal muscles; and uses as its end point 85 per cent of the age-predicted maximal heart rate (24).

In the healthy heart the changes that normally follow exercise are tachycardia, increased height of P waves, shortened P-R interval, slight ST depression—not more than 0.5 mm. and often consisting of J-point depression with progressively rising ST segment—and increased height of some T waves with inversion of others. None of these changes must be accepted as evidence of a positive exercise test. Extrasystoles frequently develop at the height of a positive test, and may be considered an integral part of the

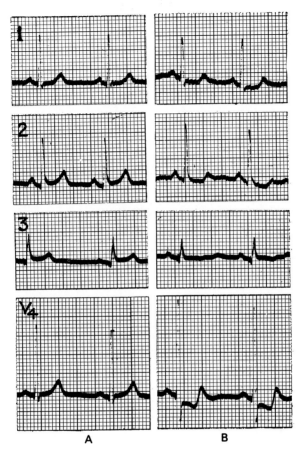

FIG. 215. **Positive exercise test.** A. Control tracing before
exercise: within normal limits. B. Two minutes after exercise:
striking ST depression in V$_4$ with lesser ST-T changes in 1
and 2.

abnormal response (fig. 214), but in themselves they are not necessarily a
sign of heart disease (11).

The anoxia test has certain advantages over the exercise test: it is usable
in patients who cannot exercise, the patient is under continuous electrocardiographic observation, oxygen is instantly available and the test immediately reversible, and the records are better because of the lack of muscle
tremor following exertion (4).

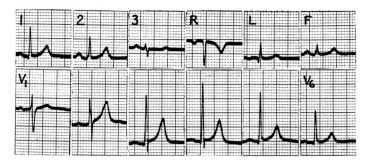

FIG. 216. Normal tracing in a patient with previous myocardial infarction and subsequent angina of effort.

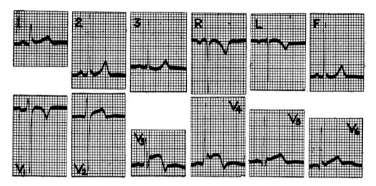

FIG. 217. From a normal Negro man of 24 years. Note marked ST elevation and T-wave inversion in V_3 and V_4.

Finally, the presence of coronary disease is *not excluded* by a normal tracing (17). The diagnosis of angina is made primarily from the history. Figure 216 is the tracing from a 42-year-old man who had a proved myocardial infarction two years previously and who has suffered from angina of effort since then. The electrocardiogram is within normal limits.

ELECTROCARDIOGRAPHOGENIC DISEASE

Abnormalities in the electrocardiogram do not necessarily indicate cardiac disease, much less coronary disease (31, 35–41). When deviations from the normal, especially those affecting the ST segments and T waves, are encountered in the middle-aged and elderly, they are much too glibly interpreted as "coronary insufficiency." Statistically such inferences are no doubt often right, but the habit is bad practice and is scientifically unsound; too many people are limping their ways through life maimed by the unkind cuts of electrocardiographic interpretation (43). Remember the following facts before attaching the "cardiac" or "coronary" label:

1. **The range of normal is wide and its limits cannot be satisfactorily defined** (49). Changes well outside the accepted range are undoubtedly at times normal variants. Examples of this are the persistent "juvenile" precordial pattern particularly seen in healthy young Negroes (30, 32) (fig. 217), unusual S-T elevation (fig. 218), also especially common in Negroes (fig. 217) (51), apparent ST depression due to carryover of T_P wave (53), ST-T

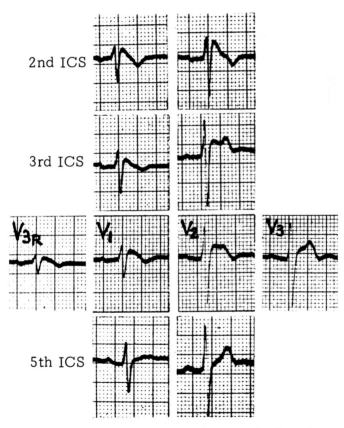

FIG. 218. Saddle-shaped, step-like and plateau elevations of precordial ST segments from a healthy dentist of 32 years. Notice the variation from interspace to interspace; thus misplacement of the electrode from day to day may trap the unwary into thinking that "evolution" is occurring.

depression in "suspended" hearts (29) (fig. 219), precordial T-wave inversion during pregnancy, prolonged P-R intervals in occasional healthy hearts (34, 47) and a right bundle-branch block pattern in marathon runners (25), whose cardiovascular competence can hardly be questioned.

2. **Numerous extracardiac factors can produce patterns similar to those seen in myocardial disease.** Without necessarily impairing cardiac competence, many factors can cause changes in the repolarization processes of the ventricles which are reflected in the electrocardiogram in T-wave or ST-segment alterations. The T wave and to a lesser extent the ST segment are unstable members that are easily upset by a great variety of major and minor provocations. Among the many stimuli that can affect them are eating (44, 46, 50), drinking ice water (28), posture (47), hyperventilation (54); emotional disturbances such as the startle reaction, fear or anxiety (33, 42) and neurocirculatory asthenia (48); numerous drugs, including digitalis, quinidine, procaine amide, adrenaline, isuprel, insulin; extracardiac diseases such as electrolyte imbalances, the acute abdomen, shock, hiatal hernia, gall bladder disease, cerebrovascular accidents (26), psychosis and endocrine disturbances.

3. Finally **the heart may be the victim of a disease that is not primarily cardiac, let alone coronary.** Pulmonary embolism, anemia, hypothyroidism, myocarditis (27) from infections (e.g., pneumonia, infectious mononucleosis), sarcoidosis, hemochromatosis, primary amyloidosis, beriberi, scleroderma, disseminated lupus, Friedreich's ataxia, progressive muscular dystrophy and myasthenia gravis all may produce changes in the tracing indicative of myocardial involvement and quite indistinguishable from some of the alterations resulting from coronary disease.

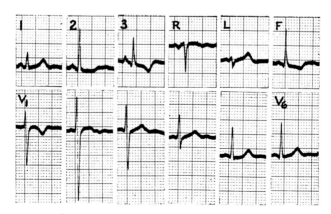

Fig. 219. Abnormal ST-T pattern in leads 2, 3 and aVF in a young woman with a "suspended" heart but no cardiac disease.

Therefore in assessing the tracing that does not conform with our accepted standards we should remember the whole array of common and uncommon possibilities and we should ask ourselves three questions: 1) Could this be a normal variant? 2) Could these abnormalities be due to extracardiac factors, physiological or pathological? and 3) Could these changes be due to heart disease other than coronary?

The danger of attributing changes of the first and second category to heart disease is that the patient is branded as a cardiac. The danger of labelling the third group as "coronary" is that the physician in charge of the case may be thereby blinded to the true nature of the cardiac involvement and of the underlying primary disease. We should often be content to state that the pattern is abnormal but non-specific. We should also certainly be at pains to spread the gospel that AN "ABNORMAL" TRACING DOES NOT NECESSARILY MEAN AN ABNORMAL HEART.

In many ways this is the most important section of this book. For if the lesson that it attempts to teach is well learned, it may save numerous people from cardiac invalidism. The whole subject of "coronary mimicry" in the electrocardiogram was reviewed elsewhere (35) with detailed discussion and a full bibliography.

REFERENCES

CORONARY INSUFFICIENCY

1. Bellet, S., et al.: Radioelectrocardiography during exercise in patients with angina pectoris. Comparison with the postexercise electrocardiogram. Circulation 1962: **25,** 5.
2. Blackburn, H., and Katigbak, R.: What electrocardiographic leads to take after exercise? Am. Heart J. 1964: **67,** 184.
3. Blackburn, H., et al.: The exercise ECG test. At what intervals to record after exercise. Am. Heart J. 1964: **67,** 186.
4. Coulshed, N.: The anoxia test for myocardial ischemia. Brit. Heart J. 1960: **22,** 79.
5. Evans, W., and McRae, C.: The lesser electrocardiographic signs of cardiac pain. Brit. Heart J. 1952: **14, 429.**
6. Fagin, I. D., and Guidot, J. M.: Post-extrasystolic T wave changes. Am. J. Cardiol. 1958: **1,** 597.
7. Gazes, P. C., et al.: The diagnosis of angina pectoris. Am. Heart J. 1964: **67,** 830.
8. Georgopoulos, A. J., et al.: Effect of exercise on electrocardiogram of patients with low serum potassium. Circulation 1961: **23,** 567.
9. Hellerstein, H. K., et al.: Two step exercise test as a test of cardiac function in chronic rheumatic heart disease and in arteriosclerotic heart disease with old myocardial infarction. Am. J. Cardiol. 1961: **7,** 234.
10. Lachman, A. B., et al.: Postural ST-T wave changes in the radioelectrocardiogram simulating myocardial ischemia. Circulation 1965: **31,** 557.
11. Lamb, L. E., and Hiss, R. G.: Influence of exercise on premature contractions. Am. J. Cardiol. 1962: **10,** 209.
12. Lepeschkin, E., and Surawicz, B.: Characteristics of true-positive and false-positive results of ECG Master two step exercise tests. New Eng. J. Med. 1958: **258,** 511.
13. Lepeschkin, E.: Exercise tests in the diagnosis of coronary heart disease. Circulation 1960: **22,** 986.

14. Levine, H. D., Lown, B., and Streeper, R. B.: The clinical significance of post-extrasystolic T wave changes. Circulation 1952: **6**, 538.

15. Lloyd-Thomas, H. G.: The effect of exercise on the electrocardiogram in healthy subjects. Brit. Heart J. 1961: **23**, 260.

16. Mann, R. H., and Burchell, H. B.: The sign of T-wave inversion in sinus beats following ventricular extrasystoles. Am. Heart J. 1954: **47**, 504.

17. Martinez-Rios, M. A., et al.: Normal electrocardiogram in the presence of severe coronary artery disease. Am. J. Cardiol. 1970: **25**, 320.

18. Meyer, P., and Herr, R.: L'intéret du syndrome éléctrocardiographique TV1 > TV6 pour le dépistage précoce de troubles de la repolarisation ventriculaire gauche. Arch. Mal. Coeur 1959: **52**, 753.

19. Prinzmetal, M., et al.: Variant form of angina pectoris. J.A.M.A. 1960: **174**, 1794.

20. Robb, G. P., and Marks, H. H.: Latent coronary artery disease. Determination of its presence and severity by the exercise electrocardiogram. Am. J. Cardiol. 1964: **13**, 603.

21. Roman, L., and Bellet, S.: Significance of the QX/QT ratio and the QT ratio (QTr) in the exercise electrocardiogram. Circulation 1965: **32**, 435.

22. Scherf, D., and Schaffer, A. I.: The electrocardiographic exercise test. Am. Heart J. 1952: **43**, 927.

23. Scherf, D.: Development of the electrocardiographic exercise test. Standardized versus non-standardized test. Am. J. Cardiol. 1960: **5**, 433.

24. Sheffield, L. T., et al.: Exercise graded by heart rate in electrocardiographic testing for angina pectoris. Circulation 1965: **32**, 622.

ELECTROCARDIOGRAPHOGENIC DISEASE

25. Beckner, G. L., and Winsor, T.: Cardiovascular adaptations to prolonged physical effort. Circulation 1954: **9**, 835.

26. Burch, G. E., Meyers, R., and Abildskov, J. A.: A new electrocardiographic pattern observed in cerebrovascular accidents. Circulation 1954: **9**, 719.

27. de la Chapelle, C. E., and Kossmann, C. E.: Myocarditis. Circulation 1954: **10**, 747.

28. Dowling, C. V., and Hellerstein, H. K.: Factors influencing the T wave of the electrocardiogram. II. Effects of drinking ice water. Am. Heart J. 1951: **41**, 58.

29. Evans, W., and Lloyd-Thomas, H. G.: The syndrome of the suspended heart. Brit. Heart J. 1957: **19**, 153.

30. Grusin, H.: Peculiarities of the African's electrocardiogram and the changes observed in serial studies. Circulation 1954: **9**, 860.

31. Levine, H. D.: Non-specificity of the electrocardiogram associated with coronary artery disease. Am. J. Med. 1953: **15**, 344.

32. Littmann, D.: Persistence of the juvenile pattern in the precordial leads of healthy adult Negroes, with report of electrocardiographic survey on three hundred Negro and two hundred white subjects. Am. Heart J. 1946: **32**, 370.

33. Magendantz, H., and Shortsleeve, J.: Electrocardiographic abnormalities in patients exhibiting anxiety. Am. Heart J. 1951: **42**, 849.

34. Manning, G. W.: Electrocardiography in the selection of Royal Canadian Air Force Aircrew. Circulation 1954: **10**, 401.

35. Marriott, H. J. L.: Coronary mimicry: normal variants, and physiologic, pharmacologic and pathologic influences that simulate coronary patterns in the electrocardiogram. Ann. Int. Med. 1960: **52**, 411.

36. Marriott, H. J. L.: Electrocardiographogenic suicide and lesser crimes. J. Florida Med. Assoc. 1963: **50**, 440.

37. Marriott, H. J. L.: Normal electrocardiographic variants simulating ischemic heart disease. J.A.M.A. 1967: **199**, 103.

38. Marriott, H. J. L., and Nizet, P. M.: Physiologic stimuli simulating ischemic heart disease. J.A.M.A. 1967: **200**, 715.
39. Marriott, H. J. L., and Menendez, M. M.: Noncoronary disease simulating myocardial ischemia or infarction. J.A.M.A. 1967: **201**, 53.
40. Marriott, H. J. L.: Dangers in overinterpretation of the electrocardiogram. Heart Bull. 1967: **18**, 61.
41. Marriott, H. J. L., and Slonim, R.: False patterns of myocardial infarction. Heart Bull. 1967: **16**, 71.
42. Mitchell, J. H., and Shapiro, A. P.: The relationship of adrenalin and T wave changes in the anxiety state. Am. Heart J. 1954: **48**, 323.
43. Prinzmetal, M., et al.: Clinical implications of errors in electrocardiographic interpretations: heart disease of electrocardiographic origin. J.A.M.A. 1956: **161**, 138.
44. Rochlin, I., and Edwards, W. L. J.: The misinterpretation of electrocardiograms with postprandial T-wave inversion. Circulation 1954: **10, 843**.
45. Roesler, H.: An electrocardiographic study of high takeoff of R (R')-T segment in right precordial leads. Altered repolarization. Am. J. Cardiol. 1960: **6**, 920.
46. Sears, G. A., and Manning, G. W.: Routine electrocardiography: postprandial T-wave changes. Am. Heart J. 1958: **56**, 591.
47. Scherf, D., and Dix, J. H.: The effects of posture on A-V conduction. Am. Heart J. 1952: **43**, 494.
48. Silverman, J. J., and Goodman, R. D.: Extraordinary alteration of P-R interval in neurocirculatory asthenia. Am. Heart J. 1951: **41**, 155.
49. Simonson, E.: Editorial: Principles for determination of electrocardiographic normal standards. Am. Heart J. 1956: **52**, 163.
50. Simonson, E., and Keys, A.: The effect of an ordinary meal on the electrocardiogram. Normal standards in middle aged men and women. Circulation 1950: **1**, 1000.
51. Thomas, J., Harris, E., and Lassiter, G.: Observations on the T wave and S-T segment changes in the precordial electrocardiogram of 320 young Negro adults. Am. J. Cardiol. 1960: **5**, 468.
52. Wasserburger, R. H., and Alt, W. J.: The normal RS-T segment elevation variant. Am. J. Cardiol. 1961: **8**, 184.
53. Wasserburger, R. H., et al.: The T-a wave of the adult electrocardiogram: an expression of pulmonary emphysema. Am. Heart J. 1957: **54**, 875.
54. Wasserburger, R. H., Siebecker, K. L., and Lewis, W. C.: The effect of hyperventilation on the normal adult electrocardiogram. Circulation 1956: **13**, 850.

Review Tracing

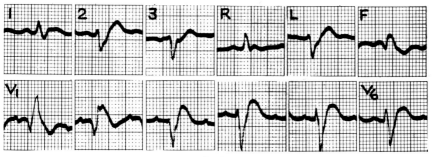

TR-31

For interpretation, see pages 314–17

Review Tracings

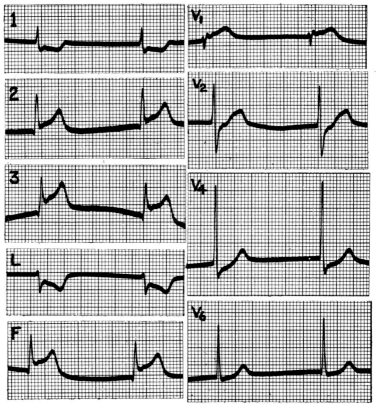

TR-32

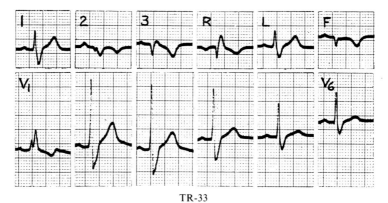

TR-33

For interpretation, see pages 314–17

Review Tracing

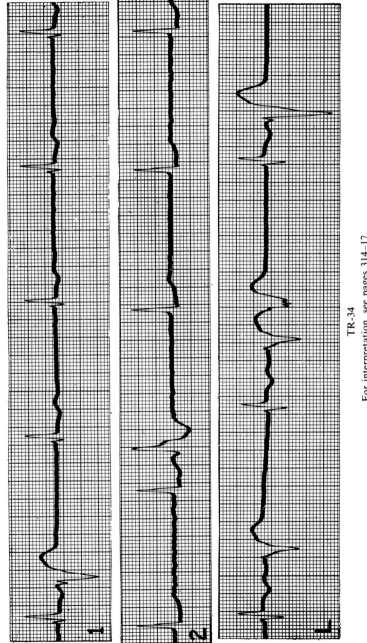

TR-34

For interpretation, see pages 314-17

20

The Heart in Childhood and Congenital Lesions

Several points are of importance in interpreting the electrocardiogram in children. First and foremost, variations in the normal are more diverse than they are in adult tracings, so that one should be even more careful in declaring a youthful tracing abnormal than that of an adult. The rate is relatively faster, and the P-R and QRS intervals relatively shorter in childhood.

At birth the right ventricular wall is almost as thick as that of the left, and this leads to a different balance of power. Apart from the common occurrence of right axis deviation, tall R waves are frequently seen in precordial leads to the right of the precordium with deep S waves in left chest leads. Thus a pattern resembling right ventricular hypertrophy or right bundle-branch block in the adult may be a perfectly normal finding in the child.

A further important point to remember is that T waves may be normally inverted further to the left of the precordium in the child (see page 24). The percentage of incidence of T-wave inversion in the first four chest leads is as follows (22, 28):

	V_1	V_2	V_3	V_4
6–12 mo	100	91	57	4.3
1–3 yr	96	77	38	4
8–12 yr	82	13.2	4.45	0

CONGENITAL HEART DISEASE

Many congenital lesions may be associated with a normal electrocardiogram. Normal tracings are more often seen in lesions that place primary stress on the left ventricle, such as aortic stenosis, coarctation of the aorta, ventricular septal defect and patent ductus; they are less often seen in association with lesions that stress the right ventricle, such as pulmonic stenosis and atrial septal defect. Complex defects are only rarely associated with a normal tracing. A normal tracing, therefore, by no means excludes a congenital lesion.

Again, there may be great differences between the tracings from different patients with the same deformity; for example, in mild patent ductus or ventricular septal defect the tracing will probably be normal. Later the pattern of left ventricular diastolic overloading may develop (fig. 220). When pulmonary hypertension becomes significant, right ventricular hypertrophy will be added to the left ventricular overloading pattern. Finally, when pulmonic hypertension is marked, the pattern may become that of right ventricular hypertrophy alone.

In congenital heart disease few patterns are diagnostic and those that are are associated with the rarer malformations: for example, when the left coronary arises from the pulmonary artery (anomalous left coronary artery), the electrocardiographic pattern is usually diagnostic—Q waves, ST elevation and T-wave inversion are present in

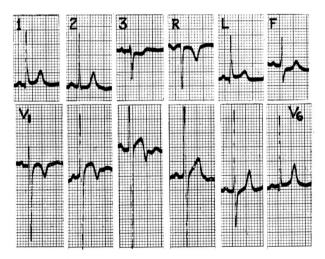

Fig. 220. From a patient with **patent ductus arteriosus,** showing left ventricular diastolic overloading. Note high voltage of QRS complexes, with tall upright T waves in V_{5-6}. U waves are inverted in 1, 2 and V_6.

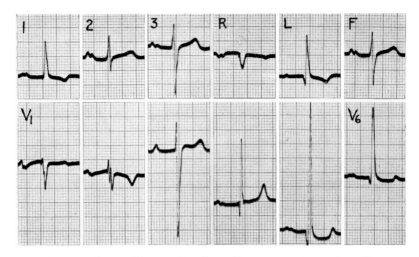

FIG. 221. From a 24-year-old patient with **patent ductus arteriosus.** Note wide notched P waves (intra-atrial block, evidence of left atrial enlargement), first degree A-V block (P-R = 0.30 sec.) and high voltage QRS complexes with ST-T changes indicating left ventricular hypertrophy and strain.

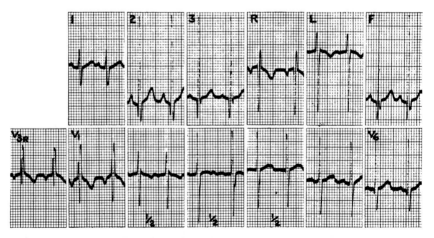

FIG. 222. From a child with **ventricular septal defect.** Note deep Q waves in 2, 3 and aVF. incomplete RBBB pattern and equiphasic RS pattern in midprecordial leads. (Reproduced from Marriott: *Bedside Diagnosis of Heart Disease*, Tampa Tracings, 1967.)

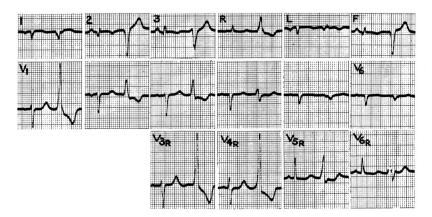

FIG. 223. From a patient with **situs inversus,** acute inferior infarction and ventricular bigeminy. Note inverted P and QRS in lead 1 and dwindling S wave across left precordium. When precordial leads are taken to the right (V_{3R}-V_{6R}), the normal transition from rS to R occurs.

leads 1, aVL and the left chest leads, giving a pattern identical with that of anterolateral infarction (13). The electrocardiogram of dextrocardia with situs inversus is also almost specific, and those of the ostium primum/common A-V canal group and Ebstein's disease are relatively so (see below). Although the tracing is seldom truly diagnostic, it often serves as a helpful guidepost and it is convenient to gather the most useful pointers under the headings of the four main components of the tracing:

P waves.

> a) In isolated dextrocardia the P wave in lead 1 is normally upright, whereas in dextrocardia with situs inversus it is inverted (left-sided venous atrium and vena cava); indeed all complexes in lead 1 are inverted (fig. 223).

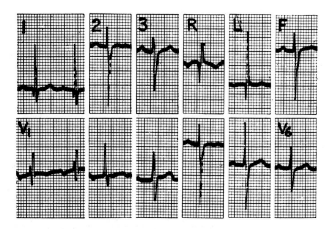

FIG. 224. From a 13-year-old boy with an **ostium primum** atrial septal defect, cleft mitral valve and small ventricular septal defect (incomplete **A-V communis**); note the almost diagnostic combination of marked left axis deviation of the early portion of the QRS (presumably due to congenital left anterior hemiblock) with incomplete RBBB.

b) **P-congenitale** consists of tall and peaked P waves in leads 1 and 2, with tall, mainly positive P waves in right chest leads (fig. 225). The frontal plane axis is generally between +30° and +45°, in contrast with one to the right of +60° in P-pulmonale. P-congenitale is found mainly in cyanotic forms of congenital disease but also in pure pulmonic stenosis. The tallest P waves occur in tricuspid disease (stenosis or atresia) and in Ebstein's disease (fig. 226).

QRS complex.

a) Determination of the **mean QRS axis** may provide a helpful initial clue to diagnosis. Diagrams illustrating the distribution of congenital malformations in the various segments of the hexaxial reference system have been published, and these may profitably be consulted (10, 15, 23). When **left axis deviation** is seen in a patient with cyanotic disease, the most likely diagnosis is tricuspid atresia; but other possibilities include transposition of the great vessels, single ventricle

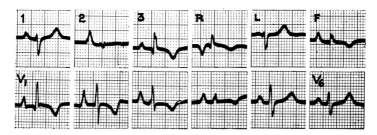

FIG. 225. From a 44-year-old patient with **pulmonic stenosis.** Tracing shows right ventricular hypertrophy and strain (systolic overloading). Note P-congenitale, indicating right atrial enlargement, with prominent R waves in right precordial leads, marked right axis deviation ($+150°$) and relatively low equiphasic complexes in V_{5-6}.

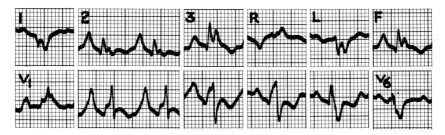

FIG. 226. **Ebstein's anomaly.** From a 36-year-old woman with severe Ebstein's anomaly. Note low voltage, atypical RBBB and enormous P waves.

and a number of other anomalies (20). When the initial portion of the QRS complex shows marked left axis deviation while the terminal part shows a right bundle-branch block, the overwhelming probability is a lesion of the ostium primum/A-V communis group (endocardial cushion defect) (fig. 224). Such a pattern is unfortunately also sometimes seen in secundum defects (14).

b) The patterns of **ventricular hypertrophy** are obviously of considerable diagnostic importance; right ventricular hypertrophy is seen in pure pulmonic stenosis (fig. 225), atrial septal defect and most of the cyanotic lesions. In the tetralogy of Fallot, the dominant R wave in V_1 of right ventricular hypertrophy usually changes to RS or rS by V_2, whereas in pure pulmonic stenosis the R wave usually remains dominant in the first 3 or 4 chest leads (fig. 225).

Left hypertrophy is seen in aortic stenosis, coarctation of the aorta, ventricular septal defect and patent ductus. In aortic stenosis, an R/T ratio of more than 10 in V_5 or V_6 indicates severe obstruction (11). Note that ventricular hypertrophy and axis deviation do not necessarily go hand in hand. Indeed, left axis deviation is seen in less than 25 per cent of cases showing left ventricular hypertrophy, and right axis deviation is present in less than 66 per cent of those showing right ventricular hypertrophy.

c) **Bundle-branch block.** Right bundle-branch block is commonly seen as a hemodynamic expression of right ventricular diastolic overloading (fig. 227). The classic example is atrial septal defect, and up to 90 per cent of patients with this lesion manifest right bundle-branch block. It is also frequently seen in the hemodynamically similar total anomalous pulmonary venous return and turns up occasionally in a variety of other lesions. It is a well-recognized complication of surgery for ventricular septal defect (fig. 232). In Ebstein's disease right bundle-branch block is the rule, but in this condition the QRS complexes of the right precordial leads are typically of quite low voltage (fig. 226). Left bundle-branch block is rare but is occasionally seen in aortic stenosis and in other lesions placing predominant strain on the left ventricle. It regularly occurs following surgery for muscular subaortic stenosis.

d) **Pre-excitation.** The W-P-W syndrome has been described in a variety of congenital lesions, but much its commonest associations are Ebstein's anomaly and primary cardiomyopathy (17, 24).

e) The **Katz-Wachtel phenomenon** consists of equiphasic complexes in two or more limb leads, often with similar equiphasicity in the mid-precordial leads. This is seen in many congenital lesions, but is perhaps most common in ventricular septal defect (fig. 222).

f) Prominent **Q waves** in the right precordial leads are evidence of right *atrial* hypertrophy; prominent Q waves in left chest leads, or in 2, 3, and aVF, some-

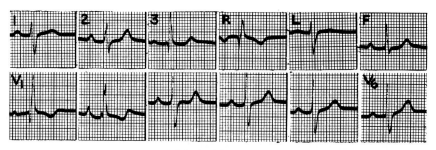

FIG. 227. **Atrial septal defect.** Typical RBBB pattern of right ventricular diastolic over-loading. Note also 1st degree A-V block and pointed right precordial P waves suggesting right atrial hypertrophy.

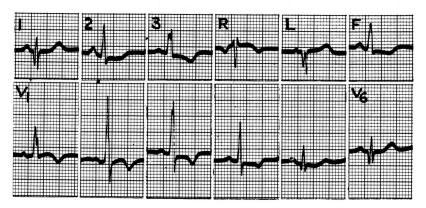

FIG. 228. **Muscular subaortic stenosis.** Note deep Q waves in 1, aVL and V_6, with reciprocal tall R in right chest leads, indicating septal hypertrophy.

times reaching a depth of 10 mm., are most suspicious of ventricular septal defect (figs. 222 and 232). Prominent Q waves in limb and left chest leads are also typical of muscular subaortic stenosis (fig. 228).

T waves.

In differentiating Fallot's tetralogy from the trilogy (pulmonic stenosis, atrial septal defect and right ventricular hypertrophy) or from pure pulmonic stenosis, T-wave behavior may be helpful. In the tetralogy precordial T waves are usually inverted

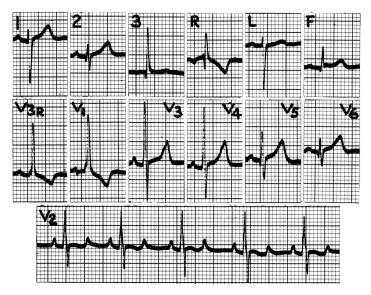

FIG. 229. **Tetralogy of Fallot.** Note marked right axis deviation (+150°) with right ventricular hypertrophy. T waves become upright in V₂ (compare with persistent inversion through V₄ in pure pulmonic stenosis—fig. 225).

only in leads taken to the right of the sternum (fig. 229), whereas in the trilogy or pure pulmonic stenosis they are frequently inverted as far to the left as V_4 or V_5 (fig. 225).

U waves.

These have been largely neglected in descriptions of the electrocardiogram in congenital heart disease; but inverted U waves are a common finding in left chest leads as an early sign of left ventricular overloading, systolic or diastolic.

INDIVIDUAL DEFECTS

The cardinal features of the electrocardiogram in the commoner congenital lesions and in those with distinctive features are as follows:

Ventricular septal defect (VSD) (figs. 222, 232)

Prominent Q waves in left chest leads or in 2, 3 and aVF. High voltage equiphasic QRS complex in mid-precordial leads in 50 to 75 per cent.

Pattern of RBBB, complete or more often incomplete, in 20 to 30 per cent.

Depending on severity and stage, may be normal, or show LVH, combined ventricular hypertrophy or RVH; LVH is often of diastolic overloading type.

Patent ductus arteriosus (figs. 220, 221)

Similar to VSD; but left atrial enlargement and 1st degree A-V block are more common and RBBB patterns less common than in VSD.

Atrial septal defect (fig. 227)

Patterns of RBBB in majority—up to 90 per cent in some series.
P-congenitale in some.
1st degree A-V block and atrial arrhythmias in a few.

Aortic stenosis

Normal in at least 25 per cent of those with significant obstruction.
Varying stages of LVH in most of remainder.
LBBB in a few.

Muscular subaortic stenosis (fig. 228)

Axis usually normal.
Delta waves are common; occasional W-P-W.
Prominent Q waves, especially in leads 2, 3, aVF, V_{5-6}; with tall R waves in right chest leads (evidence of septal hypertrophy). Progression from this to LVH.

Coarctation (fig. 230)

Normal or LVH.

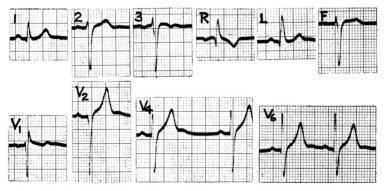

FIG. 230. From a 15-year-old boy with **coarctation of the aorta.** Note unusually marked left axis deviation $(-75°)$, presumably due to left anterior hemiblock.

Pulmonic stenosis (PS) (fig. 225)

RVH with rR or qR in V_1 when RV pressure is equal to or higher than LV pressure; Rs or rS in V_1 when RV pressure is less than LV pressure.

P-congenitale.

In severe PS, R waves dominant and T waves inverted V_1 to V_3 or V_4.

Tetralogy of Fallot (figs. 229, 232)

RVH with dominant R and inverted T in V_1, with abrupt change to rS with upright T in V_2 or V_3 (cf. pulmonic stenosis).

P-congenitale.

Transposition of great vessels

RVH with a) qR in V_1 suggests intact ventricular septum; b) rsR' in V_1 suggests VSD.

P-congenitale.

T waves taller in right than left chest leads.

Corrected transposition (fig. 231)

qR in V_1 with no q and RS in V_6.

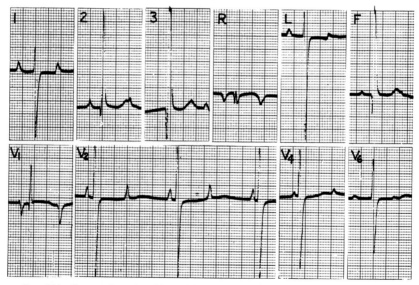

FIG. 231. **Corrected transposition** of the great vessels. Note the left ventricular (qR) pattern in V_1 with absent Q and deep S in V_6—typical of ventricular inversion; also the P-congenitale type of right atrial enlargement and the high grade (probably complete) A-V block. (Reproduced from Marriott: *Bedside Diagnosis of Heart Disease.* Tampa Tracings, 1967.)

P-congenitale.

Some degree of A-V block.

Endocardial cushion defect (fig. 224)

Left axis deviation of initial portion of QRS with incomplete RBBB pattern.

Occasional 1st degree A-V block.

Ebstein's anomaly (fig. 226)

Right atrial enlargement without RVH.

Low amplitude, atypical RBBB pattern.

W-P-W syndrome in 10 per cent.

1st degree A-V block in 15 to 20 per cent.

Arrhythmias, especially atrial tachycardia.

Tricuspid atresia

LVH, or at least left axis deviation, in 80 to 90 per cent.

P-tricuspidale.

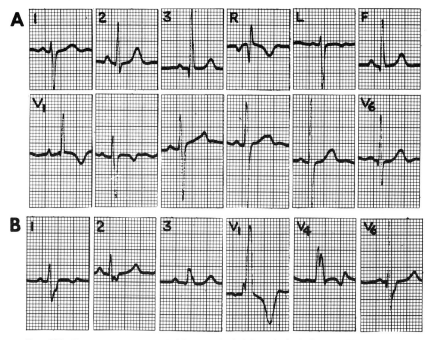

Fig. 232. **Tetralogy of Fallot.** A. Note marked right axis deviation (+120°), tall R in V_1 and deep S waves through V_6; also that S waves become dominant at V_2 while T waves are upright at V_3 (compare pattern of pure pulmonic stenosis, fig. 225). B. Development of RBBB following surgical correction.

REFERENCES

1. Beregovich, J., et al.: The vectorcardiogram and electrocardiogram in persistent common atrioventricular canal. Circulation 1960: **21,** 63.
2. Beregovich, J., et al.: The vectorcardiogram and electrocardiogram in ventricular septal defect. Brit. Heart J. 1960: **22,** 205.
3. Braudo, M., et al.: A distinctive electrocardiogram in muscular subaortic stenosis due to septal hypertrophy. Am. J. Cardiol. 1964: **14,** 599.
4. Braunwald, E., et al.: Idiopathic hypertrophic subaortic stenosis. I. A description of the disease based upon an analysis of 64 patients. Circulation 1964: **30,** Supp. IV-3.
5. Brink, A. J., and Neill, C. A.: The electrocardiogram in congenital heart disease: with special reference to left axis deviation. Circulation 1955: **12,** 604.
6. Brumlik, J. V.: Principles of electrocardiographic interpretation in congenital heart disease. In *Advances in Electrocardiography*, p. 203. Grune and Stratton, New York, 1958.
7. Burchell, H. B., DuShane, J. W., and Brandenburg, R. O.: The electrocardiogram of patients with atrioventricular cushion defects (defects of the atrioventricular canal). Am. J. Cardiol. 1960: **6,** 575. .
8. Dack, S.: The electrocardiogram and vectorcardiogram in ventricular septal defect. Am. J. Cardiol. 1960: **5,** 199.
9. de Oliviera, J. M., and Zimmerman, H. A.: The electrocardiogram in interatrial septal defects and its correlation with hemodynamics. Am. Heart J. 1958: **55,** 369.
10. de Oliviera, J. M., et al.: The mean ventricular axis in congenital heart disease: a study considering the natural incidence of the malformations. Am. Heart J. 1959: **57,** 820.
11. Fowler, R. S.: Ventricular repolarization in congenital aortic stenosis. Am. Heart J. 1965: **70,** 603.
12. Grant, R. P., et al.: Symposium on diagnostic methods in the study of left-to-right shunts. Circulation 1957: **16, 791.**
13. Kuzman, W. J., et al.: Anomalous left coronary artery arising from the pulmonary artery. Am. Heart J. 1959: **57, 36.**
14. Harrison, D. C., and Morrow, A. G.: Electrocardiographic evidence of left-axis deviation in patients with defects of the atrial septum of the secundum type. New Eng. J. Med. 1963: **269,** 743.
15. Landero, C. A., et al.: The mean manifest electrical axes of ventricular activation and repolarization processes (ÂQRS and ÂT) in congenital heart disease: frontal and horizontal planes. Am. Heart J. 1959: **58,** 889.
16. Pryor, R., et al.: Electrocardiographic changes in atrial septal defects: ostium secundum defect versus ostium primum (endocardial cushion) defect. Am. Heart J. 1959: **58,** 689.
17. Schiebler, G. L., et al.: The Wolff-Parkinson-White syndrome in infants and children. Pediatrics 1959: **24,** 585.
18. Scott, R. C.: The electrocardiogram in atrial septal defects and atrioventricular cushion defects. Am. Heart J. 1961: **62,** 712.
19. Scott, R. C.: The electrocardiogram in ventricular septal defects. Am. Heart J. 1961: **62,** 842.
20. Shaher, R. M.: Left ventricular preponderance and left axis deviation in cyanotic congenital heart disease. Brit. Heart J. 1963: **25,** 726.
21. Sodi-Pallares, D., and Marsico, F.: The importance of electrocardiographic patterns in congenital heart disease. Am. Heart J. 1955: **49,** 202.
22. Sodi-Pallares, D., et al.: Electrocardiography in infants and children. Ped. Clin. North Am. 1958: **5,** 871.

23. Sodi-Pallares, D., et al.: The mean manifest electrical axis of the ventricular activation process (ÂQRS) in congenital heart disease: a new approach in electrocardiographic diagnosis. Am. Heart J. 1958: **55,** 681.

24. Swiderski, J., et al.: The Wolff-Parkinson-White syndrome in infancy and childhood. Brit. Heart J. 1962: **24,** 561.

25. Toscano-Barboza, E. M., Brandenburg, R. O., and Swan, H. J. C.: Atrial septal defect. The electrocardiogram and its hemodynamic correlation in 100 proved cases. Am. J. Cardiol. 1958: **2,** 698.

26. Toscano-Barboza, E. M., and DuShane, J. W.: Ventricular septal defect. Correlation of electrocardiographic and hemodynamic findings in 60 proved cases. Am. J. Cardiol. 1959: **3,** 721.

27. Wigle, E. D., and Baron, R. H.: The electrocardiogram in muscular subaortic stenosis. Circulation 1966: **34,** 585.

28. Ziegler, R. R.: *Electrocardiographic Studies in Normal Infants and Children.* Charles C Thomas, Springfield, Ill., 1951.

Review Tracing

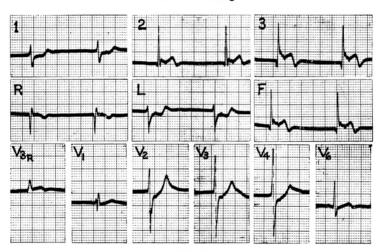

TR-35

For interpretation, see pages 314–17

Review Tracings

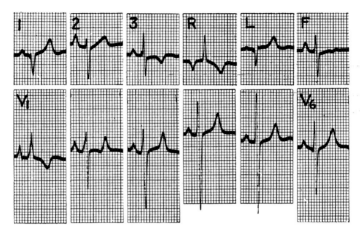

TR-36

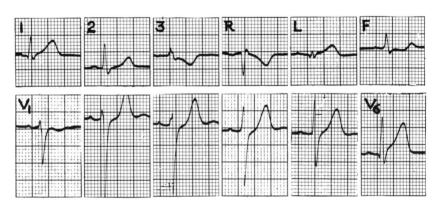

TR-37
For interpretations, see pages 314–17

Review Tracing

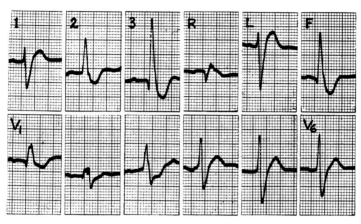

TR-38
For interpretation, see pages 314–17

21

Miscellaneous Conditions

VALVULAR LESIONS

The electrocardiogram plays only a small part in the diagnosis of valvular lesions. Mitral stenosis is the only one which may claim anything like a specific pattern (1). The **P-mitrale** pattern, consisting of wide, notched P waves in leads 1 and 2, with flat, diphasic or inverted P waves in 3, is frequently found (fig. 233). P-wave notching is sometimes best seen in mid-precordial leads (e.g., V_3). The combination of right axis deviation (with or without right ventricular hypertrophy) and the P-mitrale pattern or atrial fibrillation is strongly suggestive of mitral stenosis. The combination of right axis deviation with atrial fibrillation in a patient under 40 is practically diagnostic of mitral stenosis; but it is occasionally found in thyrotoxicosis and in atrial septal defect. The QRS voltage in lead 1 is often strikingly low (fig. 233B).

The effect of other valvular lesions can be predicted from the known mechanical effects on the heart. Aortic or mitral regurgitation predominantly affects the left ventricle and initially produces a pattern of left ventricular diastolic overloading; later they, like aortic stenosis, produce the typical pattern of left ventricular hypertrophy and strain (fig. 234).

Combined mitral and aortic lesions often produce patterns suggesting enlargement of both ventricles (fig. 235). Tricuspid stenosis is suggested when right atrial enlargement is associated with a prolonged P-R interval without preponderance of either ventricle; lead V_1 not infrequently shows a low voltage rsr' complex. Pulmonic stenosis was dealt with in the section on congenital heart disease (pages 268–279).

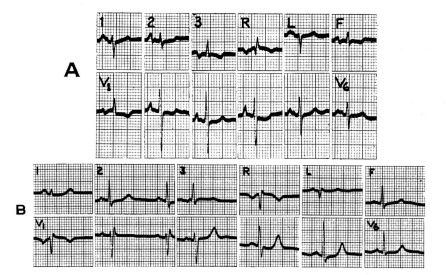

FIG. 233. A. From a patient with severe **mitral disease,** showing evidence of left atrial and right ventricular enlargement. Note P-mitrale with wide notched P waves, marked right axis deviation ($+150°$) with prominent R in V_1 and equiphasic complexes in left chest leads. B. From a 31-year-old woman with pure mitral stenosis. Note P-mitrale, low voltage QRS in lead 1 (P and R about same height) and rSr' pattern of RVH in V_{1-2}. (Reproduced from Marriott: *Bedside Diagnosis of Heart Disease.* Tampa Tracings, 1967.)

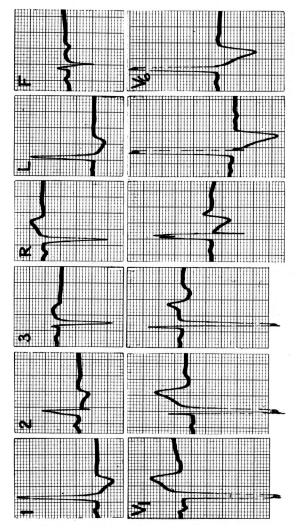

FIG. 234. From a patient with severe **syphilitic aortic insufficiency**, showing classical pattern of marked left ventricular hypertrophy and strain.

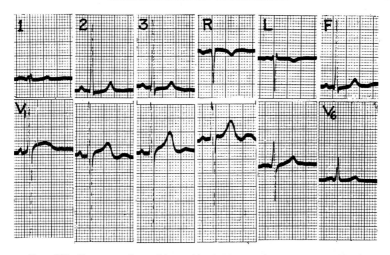

FIG. 235. From a patient with combined **mitral** and **aortic disease.** Tracing suggests biventricular hypertrophy: the high QRS voltage in 2, 3, aVF and V_{1-4} indicates left ventricular enlargement, to which the inverted U waves in 2, 3 and aVF lend supporting evidence; whereas the prominent R waves in V_{1-2}, together with the axis, which approaches $+90°$, are evidence of right ventricular hypertrophy. The flat, wide and notched P waves in 1 and V_{5-6} indicate left atrial enlargement as well.

ACUTE COR PULMONALE

The pattern of acute cor pulmonale develops rapidly, and, if the patient survives, may revert to normal within hours to a day or two, or may persist for weeks.

The pattern develops within a few minutes of a massive pulmonary embolism (4, 9) or may develop in the course of other conditions producing acute cor pulmonale (8). Its greatest importance diagnostically is that its pattern somewhat resembles that of inferior myocardial infarction, and as the clinical picture also may well be confused with myocardial infarction, the distinction is a difficult one. In the typical case, a Q wave develops in lead 3 and the ST segment becomes elevated with shallow inversion of the T wave. Meanwhile lead 1 has developed somewhat "reciprocal" changes: an S wave appears (indicating a not surprising tendency to develop right axis deviation); the ST segment is depressed while the T remains upright. All these changes are compatible with inferior infarction. Lead 2, however, tends to follow lead 1 and shows no Q wave, but an S wave, a slightly depressed ST segment and an upright T wave; whereas in inferior infarction lead 2 tends to follow lead 3 with a Q, an elevated ST and inverted T.

In the precordial leads, elevated ST segments and inverted T waves are sometimes seen over the right ventricle, while S waves may become more prominent over the left ventricle (indications of right ventricular dilation). The S wave in V_1 may become slurred and the R/S ratio decrease in two successive precordial leads (13). Transient right bundle-branch block may appear. Many of these changes are to be seen in figures 236 and 237.

The differences between this pattern and that of inferior infarction may thus be summarized as follows:

1. Lead 2 tends to follow lead 1 rather than 3.
2. The changes may be fleeting and evolve and recede in a matter of hours rather than weeks or months.
3. ST-T deviations in limb leads are slight, whereas they may be major in inferior infarction; and in right precordial leads they resemble the anteroseptal rather than the inferior infarction pattern.

A helpful aphorism: If you find yourself diagnosing inferior infarction from the limb leads, and anteroseptal damage or infarction from the chest leads, think of pulmonary embolism.

CHRONIC COR PULMONALE

Chronic cor pulmonale, most often seen in emphysema, is characterized by right axis deviation and sometimes the pattern of right ventricular hypertrophy and strain. Enlargement of the right atrium is manifested by the **P-pulmonale** pattern (fig. 238; also fig. 11, page 17), consisting of a low P in lead 1 with tall, pointed P waves in 2, 3 and aVF. The single most characteristic electrocardiographic feature of diffuse lung disease is said to be a P-wave axis between $+70°$ and $+90°$ (14). The P waves in right precordial leads are usually also pointed, or are diphasic with a distinct intrinsicoid deflection. Low voltage is not infrequently present, and T_1 is often of lower voltage than T_3.

Frequently, instead of the fullblown pattern of right ventricular hypertrophy and strain with tall R waves in V_1, an intermediate pattern is seen with deep S waves across the precordium from V_1 to V_6 (fig. 238). The Q-T interval in cor pulmonale, unlike that in other forms of heart failure, is not prolonged (3). This may at times be a helpful differential point.

The five most typical findings in emphysema (16) have been grouped together into a "pentalogy": 1) prominent P waves in 2, 3 and aVF; 2) exaggerated T_P waves producing more than 1-mm. depression of the ST segment in 2, 3 and aVF; 3) rightward shift of the QRS axis; 4) marked "clockwise rotation" in the precordial leads; and 5) low voltage of the QRS complexes, especially over the left precordium (V_{4-7}). The QRS axis in the

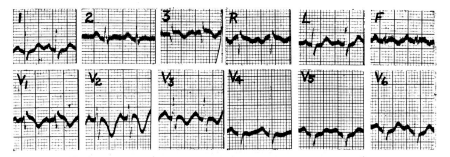

FIG. 236. **Acute cor pulmonale.** Note Q_3T_3 pattern consistent with inferior infarction, marked T-wave inversion over right precordium (V_{1-2}) and prominent S wave in 1 and 2.

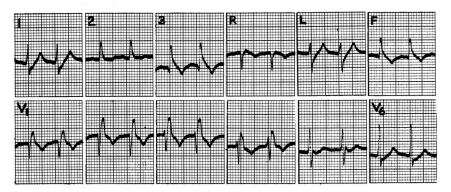

FIG. 237. **Acute cor pulmonale** (from a patient with massive pulmonary embolism). Note simultaneous inversion of T waves in inferior (3, aVF) and anteroseptal (V_{1-4}) leads, and development of RBBB.

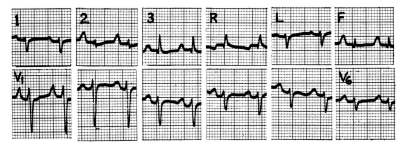

FIG. 238. **Chronic cor pulmonale.** Note P-pulmonale pattern, marked right axis shift (+150°) and deep S waves across precordium with low R waves in left chest leads.

frontal plane is sometimes in the neighborhood of $-90°$, thus simulating marked *left* axis deviation (6) (fig. 239). It is also not uncommon for Q waves simulating inferior infarction to develop in leads 2, 3 and aVF with simultaneous appearance of S waves in lead 1.

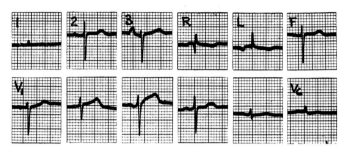

FIG. 239. From a patient with chronic lung disease. Note marked *left* axis deviation ($-60°$).

Salient Features of Chronic Cor Pulmonale

1. Right axis deviation
2. Right ventricular hypertrophy, or simply rS complexes across precordium
3. P-pulmonale pattern
4. Often low voltage QRS, and T_1 lower than T_3

ACUTE PERICARDITIS

In acute pericarditis, from whatever cause, the characteristic finding is an elevation of ST segments with upward *concavity* in many leads, including all three standard leads. The T wave remains upright at first, except in lead 3, where it may be inverted. Lead 3 is also often an exception in the shape of its ST segment, which may present an upward convexity. These changes characterize the first or **ST stage** of acute pericarditis (fig. 240).

The second stage, or **T stage,** presents widespread T-wave inversion (fig. 241). At this stage the ST segments have returned to the isoelectric level. During both stages low voltage is a common finding. In the average case of acute pericarditis resolving in the course of 3 or 4 weeks, these stages each last for about 10 days to 2 weeks.

The four most striking differences between acute pericarditis and acute infarction are tabulated in Table 3.

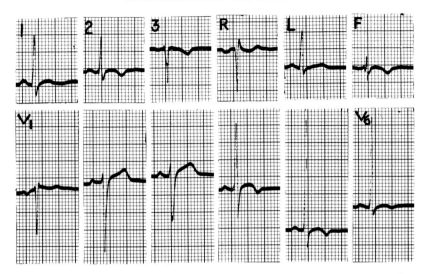

FIG. 240. **Acute pericarditis** (ST stage). Note widespread ST elevation, with upward concavity in 1, 2, aVF, and V_{4-6}.

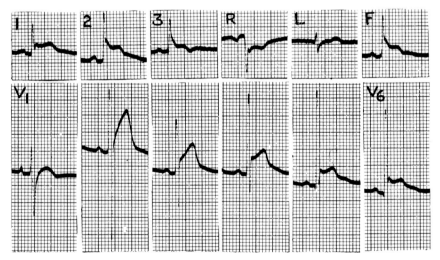

FIG. 241. **Acute pericarditis** (T stage). Note T-wave inversions in 2, 3, aVF and V_{4-6}.

The changes in pericarditis are probably due to two causes:
1. Short circuiting of impulses by pericardial fluid or thickened pericardium causes the low voltage.
2. Spread of the inflammation to the immediately subjacent layer of myocardium (i.e., subepicardial myocarditis) accounts for the ST- and T-wave changes.

TABLE 3

	Acute Pericarditis	Acute Infarction
ST reciprocity (between 1 and 3)	Absent. Elevation in both 1 and 3	Present. Elevated in one, depressed in the other
ST shape	Concave upward	Convex upward
Q waves	Absent	Present
Period of evolution	Few weeks	Months

CHRONIC CONSTRICTIVE PERICARDITIS

In the chronic constrictive or adhesive types of pericarditis changes in the tracing are relatively fixed and non-progressive. They are not unlike the findings in the T stage of the acute disease, two of the most characteristic features being low voltage and inverted T waves. Flat or inverted T waves are present in all cases, abnormal P waves in about three quarters of the cases and low voltage in over half (18).

Such changes are found in the three standard leads and in all or many of the other leads. It is of practical importance to note the degree of inversion of the T waves, for the depth of inversion is usually proportional to the degree of pericardial adherence to the myocardium (19); deep T waves are associated with intimate adherence, which makes surgical stripping difficult or impossible, whereas flat or barely inverted T waves usually indicate a relatively easy surgical undertaking.

Atrial fibrillation is persistently present in over a third of the cases (18).

One other characteristic which deserves passing mention is that the axis of the heart does not alter, as it does in the normal, when the patient turns from one side to the other; for being bound by adhesions it is not free to swing from side to side with change in position. This electrocardiographic feature corresponds with the clinical finding of a fixed apex beat.

PERICARDIAL EFFUSION

A triad that is virtually diagnostic of pericardial effusion is: low voltage, S-T segment elevation and electrical alternans (fig. 242). Total alternans, i.e., alternation of P waves as well as QRS, is almost pathognomonic and usually indicates effusion due to malignancy (17, 21).

Salient Features of Chronic Pericarditis

1. Low voltage
2. Flat or inverted T waves
3. Fixed axis
4. Possible P-mitrale pattern or atrial fibrillation

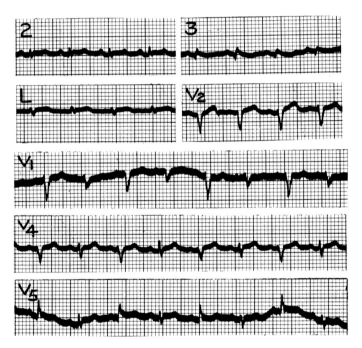

FIG. 242. **Pericardial effusion.** Note low voltage and electrical alternans of the QRS.

DIGITALIS AND THE ELECTROCARDIOGRAM

Digitalis *is* to the electrocardiogram what syphilis *was* to medicine—the great imitator. It can mimic heart disease and it can cause all types of block and all manner of arrhythmias. It is convenient to divide the effects of digitalis into four groups:

1. *ST-T changes:* digitalis causes depression of the ST segments with flattening and inversion of T waves. At the same time the relative Q-T duration is shortened in contrast to quinidine effect (see below). The shape of the depressed segment is often characteristic— sagging, with its concavity upward, and has been said to look as though a finger had been hooked over it to drag it down (figs. 243 and 244). These are not indications of digitalis *intoxication* but rather of simple digitalis *effect* unless they occur in leads with predominantly negative QRS deflections (see below). They may be anticipated in most patients who are approaching adequate digitalization and are not necessarily an indication for reducing dosage. These changes occur in animals with approximately 25 per cent of the lethal dose.

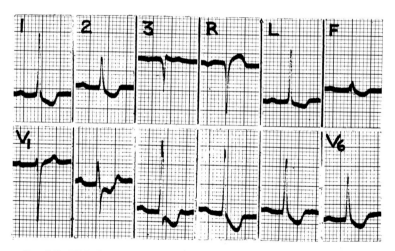

FIG. 243. **Digitalis effect.** Note sagging ST segments in most leads with short Q-T interval.

ST depression and inversion of T waves usually occur only in those leads with tall R waves. It is claimed that such displacement of ST segments and T waves in the direction opposite to the main QRS deflection means a uniform therapeutic action on the myocardium, but that depression of ST and inversion of T also in leads with mainly negative QRS complexes (fig. 244) indicates that the drug is causing relative coronary insufficiency in the subendocardial muscle layers, and is therefore an indication to reduce the dose.

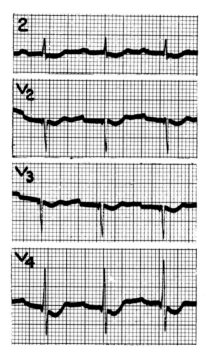

FIG. 244. **Digitalis effect.** Note sagging ST segments, even in leads that have negative QRS complexes; also short Q-T interval and first degree A-V block (P-R = 0.26 sec.).

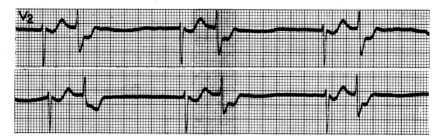

FIG. 245. **Digitalis intoxication.** Note 1) atrial fibrillation with regular independent idio-nodal rhythm, 2) ventricular bigeminy with multiform ectopic QRS complexes and 3) ST sagging in a lead with negative QRS complexes.

2. *Ventricular premature beats, often multiform* and often proceeding to *bigeminal rhythm* (fig. 245). These are of course arrhythmias and as such should be classified with the other arrhythmias below. But they are so much more often encountered than any other arrhythmia, and are therefore so suggestive of digitalis action, that they deserve a category to themselves. They are a sign of definite toxicity and are an indication to revise dosage. In animals they appear after approximately 70 per cent of the lethal dose has been administered.

3. *Arrhythmias.* Almost every arrhythmia has been reported to complicate digitalis administration. Ventricular premature beats are the commonest; but their kindred more serious rhythms, ventricular tachycardia and ventricular fibrillation, have occasionally occurred. Atrial arrhythmias may also be produced, of which the most characteristic is atrial paroxysmal tachycardia with A-V block (fig. 246). When this arrhythmia is digitalis-induced the P waves characteristically remain normally directed, their rhythm is somewhat irregular and the A-V conduction ratio varies (24). Atrial premature beats and atrial fibrillation are uncommonly due to digitalis intoxication. A-V dissociation (p. 212) is sometimes produced by digitalis as a result of sinus slowing, A-V nodal acceleration or both. Remember that digitalis in small doses depresses both sinus and A-V nodes; in higher or toxic dosage it continues to depress sinus activity but enhances A-V nodal automaticity.

4. *Blocks.* Sino-atrial, atrioventricular and intraventricular blocks have all followed digitalis administration. S-A block may induce the onset of A-V nodal rhythm. Simple lengthening of the P-R interval is common and partly results from vagal stimulation (fig. 161B, page 198). In animals it is induced by about 50 per cent of the lethal dose. Higher grades of A-V block are not infrequently seen.

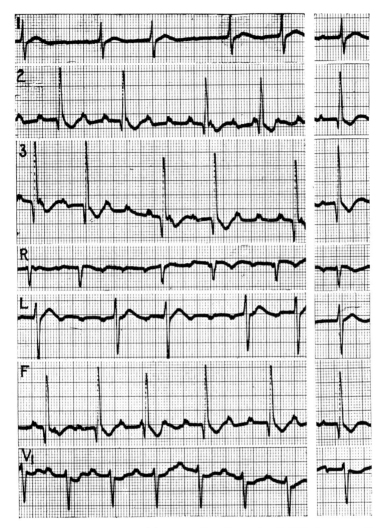

FIG. 246. Paroxysmal atrial tachycardia with varying A-V block as a result of **digitalis intoxication.** Note that the P waves are almost normally directed (axis +90°), that the A-V conduction ratio varies and that the atrial rhythm is not precisely regular. The single column of complexes on the right is to show for comparison the form and direction of P waves (axis +60°) when sinus rhythm was restored.

Complete A-V block may develop without any warning symptoms in a patient maintained on digitoxin; such block in animals indicates about 80 per cent of the lethal dose. Prolongation of the QRS interval occurs rarely in digitalis intoxication.

Slowing of the heart in sinus rhythm is not due to heart block but to enhanced vagal effect on the S-A node. In atrial fibrillation slowing of the ventricle is the desirable result of A-V block.

QUINIDINE

In general quinidine causes qualitatively similar but quantitatively different changes in the tracing. The noticeable exception to this general statement is its effect on the Q-T interval, which it regularly lengthens in contrast to digitalis effect. It is less likely to cause lengthening of the P-R interval but much more likely to prolong the QRS. Its influences may be summarized as follows:

1. *ST-T changes.* T waves become depressed, widened, notched and finally inverted. Meanwhile the Q-T interval lengthens (fig. 247). The ST segment is less likely to become depressed than with digitalis administration.
2. *Blocks* of all types can occur. S-A block may produce fatal atrial standstill. Prolongation of the QRS is frequently seen and is important to the therapist: if this interval increases during treatment by 25 to 50 per cent, it is an indication to discontinue the drug.
3. *Ventricular ectopic rhythms* are occasionally produced.

The combined effects of digitalis and quinidine (fig. 248) can closely mimic the pattern of hypokalemia (32) (see figs. 251 and 252).

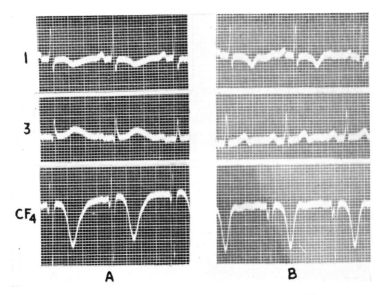

FIG. 247. **Quinidine effect.** Note the markedly prolonged Q-T interval in A of about 0.54 sec. (upper limit of normal in a male at this rate, 72, is 0.395 sec.); quinidine effect has "pulled apart" the limbs of the inverted coronary T waves in CF$_4$. In B the Q-T interval has returned to normal (0.36 sec.). Quinidine had been administered for 2 weeks before tracing A; it was discontinued on the day of this tracing, and tracing B was taken 1 week later.

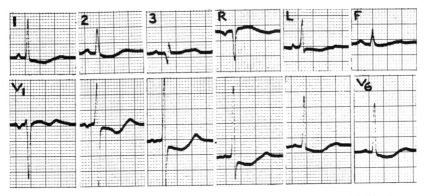

FIG. 248. **Digitalis plus quinidine effects** producing a pattern indistinguishable from that of hypokalemia (see page 302).

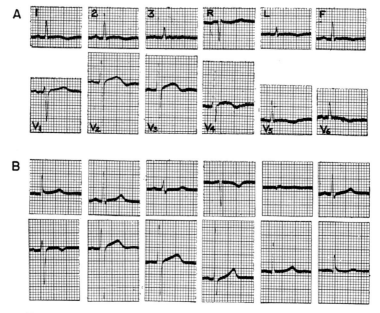

FIG. 249. **Myxedema.** Tracing A was taken before treatment; note shallow inversion of T waves in many leads. B was taken after 10 weeks of treatment with thyroid extract; the previously inverted T waves are now upright.

MYXEDEMA

The diagnosis of myxedema should certainly never depend upon electrocardiographic changes though it may be suspected when flattening or shallow inversion of many T waves is seen without comparable ST displacement (fig. 249). Its characteristics are three:

1. Low voltage
2. Sinus bradycardia (uncommon)
3. Low to inverted T waves in all or many leads

HYPOTHERMIA

When the body temperature falls below 30°C, characteristic changes develop in the electrocardiogram (fig. 250). All intervals—R-R, P-R, QRS and Q-T—may lengthen, and elevated "J deflections" appear especially in left chest leads. Atrial fibrillation may develop at about 29°C (34).

HYPOKALEMIA

The electrocardiogram may be of great value in the diagnosis of this not uncommon and dangerous situation. A significant potassium deficit may

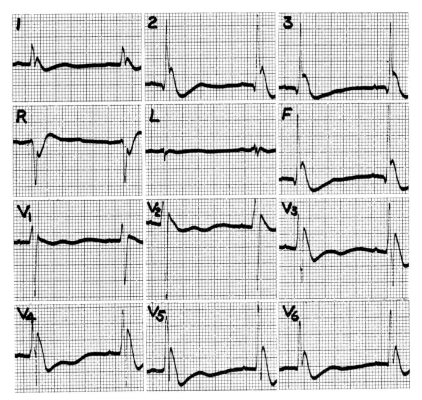

FIG. 250. **Hypothermia.** Note marked elevation of the "J deflection" maximal in mid-precordial leads.

be encountered in many metabolic disorders, including cirrhosis of the liver, diabetic coma after vigorous treatment, hypochloremic alkalosis from whatever cause (vomiting, diuresis, etc.) and in situations where excessive amounts of corticosteroids are being secreted (Cushing's syndrome, primary aldosteronism) or administered. The typical signs of potassium lack in the tracing may appear when the serum potassium is within normal limits, and conversely the tracing may be normal and show no evidence of potassium deficiency when hypokalemia is chemically proven. As the heart is most dangerously affected by too much or too little potassium, it may well be that the electrocardiogram is the most sensitive indicator of the immediate threat to life. Furthermore, an electrocardiogram can often be taken when facilities for serum determinations are not available. It is

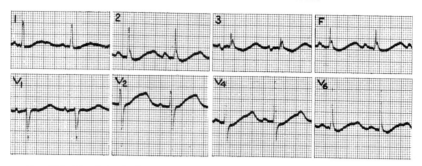

FIG. 251. **Hypokalemia.** Note characteristic pattern with ST depression and extremely prominent U waves.

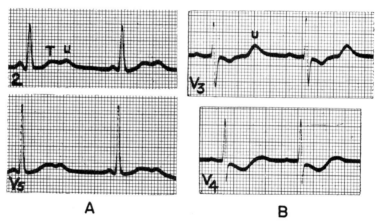

FIG. 252. **Hypokalemia.** Tracings A and B are from different patients. A shows early changes of hypokalemia with prominent U wave merging to form continuous undulating wave with T wave. B shows changes of advanced hypokalemia (1.8 mEq. per liter) in a patient with cirrhosis; note ST-T depression with very prominent U waves in V_3.

therefore worth while to know the changes that a potassium deficit can initiate (figs. 251 and 252). These usually occur in the following sequence:

1. Apparent prolongation of the Q-T interval. (This appears to be due to flattening and widening of the T wave, but more careful analysis shows that it is due to a lower T wave and taller U wave merging to form a continuous wide wave; this early stage is shown in figure 252 A.)

2. T-wave inversion

3. Sagging ST segment and finally a low "take-off" of this segment

The fully developed pattern is seen in figure 252 B. These changes rapidly revert to normal with administration of potassium salts.

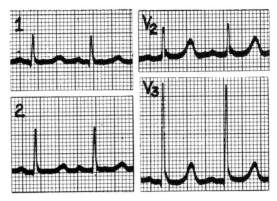

FIG. 253. **Hypocalcemia.** Note the prolonged Q-T interval in an otherwise normal tracing. Q-T = 0.40 sec. (upper limit of normal for this rate and sex is 0.35 sec.). Patient's serum calcium was 7.0 mg. per 100 ml., other electrolytes being normal.

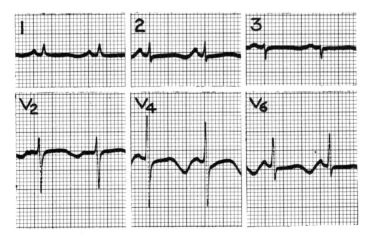

FIG. 254. **Hypocalcemia.** Note prolonged ST and QT with late inversion of T waves. From a patient with serum calcium of 4.2 mg. per 100 ml.

HYPOCALCEMIA

Calcium deficiency produces a prolonged Q-T interval. This lengthening is effected through elongation of the ST segment, the T wave remaining relatively normal (fig. 253); terminal T-wave inversion, however, occurs in some leads in about a third of the cases (fig. 254).

HYPERKALEMIA

The earliest sign of potassium intoxication is the appearance of tall, thin T waves (fig. 255). Later the P-R interval becomes prolonged, the ST segment becomes depressed and the QRS interval lengthens. Finally the P waves disappear and the QRS widens further (fig. 256) until ventricular fibrillation closes the picture. Disappearance of the P waves does not necessarily indicate a cessation of S-A node activity; despite atrial paralysis, sinus impulses may proceed to the A-V junction via specialized "internodal" conducting tracts without writing P waves, and thence onward to control the ventricles (**sinoventricular rhythm**) (29).

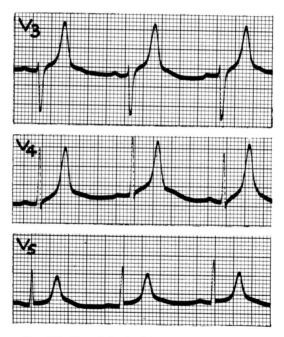

Fig. 255. **Hyperkalemia.** Note tall, pointed, "pinch-bottomed" T waves. (K = 6.1 mEq. per liter.)

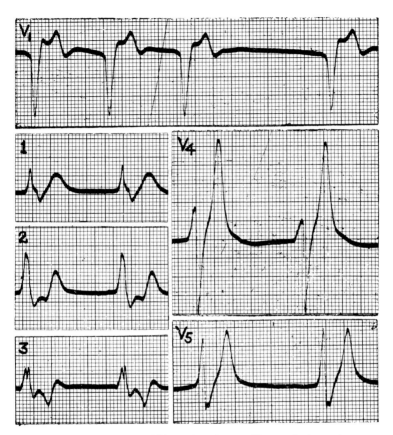

FIG. 256. **Hyperkalemia.** This tracing shows evidence of advanced potassium intoxication: tall peaked T waves, absent P waves, widened QRS complexes and irregular rhythm. From a patient with serum potassium level of 8.1 mEq. per liter.

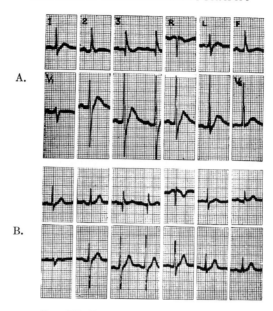

FIG. 257. From a patient with **hyperparathyroidism.** A. Before parathyroidectomy (serum calcium 15 mg.). Note virtual absence of ST segment, early peak of T wave and relatively gradual downslope of descending limb of T wave. B. After parathyroidectomy (serum calcium 10.7 mg.). Note normal contour of ST-T pattern. (Reproduced from Beck and Marriott: The electrocardiogram in hyperparathyroidism. Am. J. Cardiol. 1959: **3,** 411.)

HYPERCALCEMIA

The most striking change in the electrocardiogram is a shortening of the Q-T interval, but particularly of the distance from the beginning of the QRS to the *apex* of the T wave (Q-aT interval). This change gives the proximal limb of the T wave an abrupt slope to its peak that is most characteristic (fig. 257 A). In some cases the P-R interval is prolonged.

ELECTRICAL ALTERNANS

This abnormality is readily recognized by the alternating amplitude of QRS complexes in any or all leads (fig. 258). It is much less common than, but has the same prognostic significance as, its mechanical counterpart, *pulsus alternans*. Electrical alternans is an important part of the pattern of pericardial effusion (36) (see page 292).

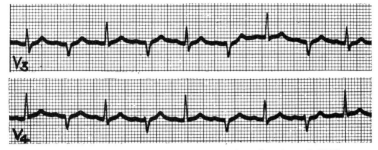

FIG. 258. **Electrical alternans.** Note alternating direction of QRS complexes.

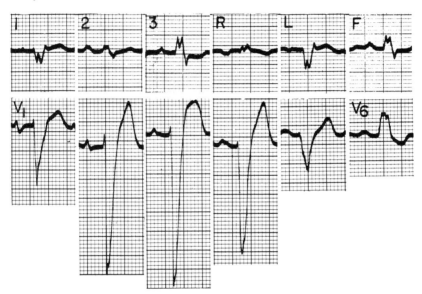

FIG. 259. **Primary cardiomyopathy.** Note the atypical pattern of intraventricular block with notching and slurring of the QRS in limb leads. P waves are also wide and notched with evidence of left atrial enlargement.

T-wave (35) and U-wave (37) alternation, without associated alternation of the QRS, have been described.

CARDIOMYOPATHY

Any electrocardiographic abnormality may accompany a cardiomyopathy (41), and none is diagnostic, with the possible exception of the progressive pattern—from septal hypertrophy (see fig. 228) to generalized LVH—seen in the prolonged follow-up of hypertrophic subaortic stenosis (38). There are, however, a few tendencies worth noting: a BBB pattern tends to be atypical and splintered (fig. 259); the association of the preexci-

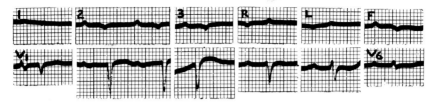

FIG. 260. **Primary amyloidosis.** Note low voltage, marked left axis deviation (of what's left of the QRS), QS complexes V_{1-3} and abnormal P waves. (Reproduced from Marriott: Correlations of electrocardiographic and pathologic changes, chapter XX in Gould's Pathology of the heart, Charles C Thomas, 2nd ed., Springfield, Ill., 1968.)

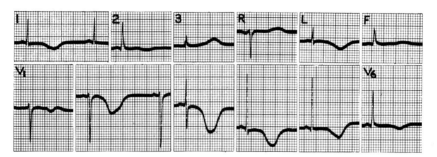

FIG. 261. **Intracerebral hemorrhage.** Note bradycardia, large inverted precordial T and U waves.

tation syndrome with familial cardiomyopathy, obstructive or nonobstructive; the combination of *left* ventricular with *right* atrial hypertrophy in muscular subortic stenosis (40); the dearth of significant arrhythmia or block in obstructive cardiomyopathy; and the tendency to *right* ventricular hypertrophy and *right* BBB in endomyocardial fibrosis.

In cardiac amyloidosis (39) the diagnosis may be suspected from the combination of low voltage, marked left axis deviation and QS or tiny rS complexes from V_1 to V_3 or V_4 (fig. 260).

Glycogen storage disease tends to produce oversized QRS complexes in all leads in company with a short P-R interval (42).

INTRACRANIAL HEMORRHAGE

Intracerebral or subarachnoid hemorrhage can produce dramatic changes in the electrocardiogram (43–45). Precordial T waves become wide and prominent, usually inverted but sometimes upright, and are continuous with large U waves, giving the effect of a long-drawn-out T-U complex (fig. 261). Bradycardia frequently accompanies these changes.

LOW VOLTAGE WITH INVERTED T WAVES

It is opportune to review the several conditions which can cause low voltage QRS with inverted T waves in all or most leads:
1. Any diffuse myocardial involvement
    a. Diffuse ischemic disease
    b. Heart failure treated with digitalis
    c. Myxedema
    d. Cardiomyopathy
2. Pericarditis
    a. Acute ("T stage")
    b. Chronic constrictive

ST-T DEPRESSION

When ST segments are depressed and T waves flat to inverted in many leads, one should think of:
1. Digitalis effect
2. Diffuse ischemic disease
3. Left ventricular strain
4. Combined anterior and inferior infarction (antero-inferior infarction)
5. Subendocardial infarction
6. Hypokalemia

As well as the above causes of ST-segment and T-wave changes, the many factors that can influence these labile members of the electrocardiogram (pages 260–263) should be constantly borne in mind.

REFERENCES

MITRAL DISEASE

1. Fraser, H. R. L., and Turner, R.: Electrocardiography in mitral valvular disease. Brit. Heart J. 1955: **17,** 459.
2. Demerdash, H., and Goodwin, J. F.: The cardiogram of mitral restenosis. Brit. Heart J. 1963: **25,** 474.

COR PULMONALE

3. Alexander, J. K., et al.: The Q-T interval in chronic cor pulmonale. Circulation 1951: **3,** 733.
4. Eliaser, M., and Giansiracusa, F.: The electrocardiographic diagnosis of acute cor pulmonale. Am. Heart J. 1952: **43,** 533.
5. Fowler, N. O., et al.: The electrocardiogram in cor pulmonale with and without emphysema. Am. J. Cardiol. 1965: **16,** 500.
6. Grant, R. P.: Left axis deviation. An electrocardiographic-pathologic correlation study. Circulation 1956: **14,** 233.
7. Littmann, D.: The electrocardiographic findings in pulmonary emphysema. Am. J. Cardiol. 1960: **5,** 339.
8. Mack, I., Harris, R., and Katz, L. N.: Acute cor pulmonale in the absence of pulmonary embolism. Am. Heart J. 1950: **39,** 664.

9. Phillips, E., and Levine, H. D.: A critical evaluation of extremity and precordial electrocardiography in acute cor pulmonale. Am. Heart J. 1950: **39**, 205.
10. Phillips, R. W.: The electrocardiogram in cor pulmonale secondary to pulmonary emphysema: a study of 18 cases proved by autopsy. Am. Heart J. 1958: **56**, 352.
11. Scott, R. C.: The electrocardiogram in pulmonary emphysema and chronic cor pulmonale. Am. Heart J. 1961: **61**, 843.
12. Selvester, R. H., and Rubin, H. B.: New criteria for the electrocardiographic diagnosis of emphysema and cor pulmonale. Am. Heart J. 1965: **69**, 437.
13. Smith, McK., and Ray, C. T.: Electrocardiographic signs of early right ventricular enlargement in acute pulmonary embolism. Chest 1970: **58**, 205.
14. Spodick, D. H.: Electrocardiographic studies in pulmonary disease. I. Electrocardiographic abnormalities in diffuse lung disease. Circulation 1959: **20**, 1067.
15. Wasserburger, R. H., et al.: The T-a wave of the adult electrocardiogram: an expression of pulmonary emphysema. Am. Heart J. 1957: **54**, 875.
16. Wasserburger, R. H., et al.: The electrocardiographic pentalogy of pulmonary emphysema. Circulation 1959: **20**, 831.

PERICARDIAL DISEASE

17. Bashour, F. A., and Cochran, P. W.: The association of electrical alternans with pericardial effusion. Dis. Chest 1963: **44**, 146.
18. Dalton, J. C., Pearson, R. J., and White, P. D.: Constrictive pericarditis: a review and long term follow-up of 78 cases. Ann. Int. Med. 1956: **45**, 445.
19. Evans, W., and Jackson, F.: Constrictive pericarditis. Brit. Heart J. 1952: **14**, 53.
20. Hull, E.: The electrocardiogram in pericarditis. Am. J. Cardiol. 1961: **7**, 21.
21. Nizet, P. M., and Marriott, H. J. L.: The electrocardiogram and pericardial effusion. J.A.M.A. 1966: **198**, 169.
22. Surawicz, B., and Lasseter, K. C.: Electrocardiogram in pericarditis. Am. J. Cardiol. 1970: **26, 471**.

DIGITALIS

23. Broome, R. A., Estes, E. H., and Orgain, E. S.: The effects of digitoxin upon the twelve lead electrocardiogram. Am. J. Med. 1956: **21**, 237.
24. Lown, B., et al.: Digitalis and atrial tachycardia with block. A year's experience. New England J. Med. 1959: **260**, 301.
25. Pick, A.: Digitalis and the electrocardiogram. Circulation 1957: **15**, 603.

ELECTROLYTES

26. Bellet, S.: The electrocardiogram in electrolyte imbalance. Arch. Int. Med. 1955: **96**, 618.
27. Bronsky, D., et al.: Calcium and the electrocardiogram. I. The electrocardiographic manifestations of hypoparathyroidism. Am. J. Cardiol. 1961: **7**, 823. II. The electrocardiographic manifestations of hyperparathyroidism and of marked hypercalcemia from various other etiologies. Ibid.: **7**, 833.
28. Dreyfus, L. S., and Pick, A.: A clinical correlation study of the electrocardiogram in electrolyte imbalance. Circulation 1956: **14**, 815.
29. Sherf, L., and James, T. N.: A new electrocardiographic concept: syncronized sinoventricular conduction. Dis. Chest 1969: **55**, 127.
30. Surawicz, B., and Lepeschkin, E.: The electrocardiographic pattern of hypopotassemia with and without hypocalcemia. Circulation 1953: **8**, 801.
31. Surawicz, B., et al.: Quantitative analysis of the electrocardiographic pattern of hypopotassemia. Circulation 1957: **16**, 750.

32. Surawicz, B.: Electrolytes and the electrocardiogram. Am. J. Cardiol. 1963: **12,** 656.
33. Weaver, W. F., and Burchell, H. B.: Serum potassium and the electrocardiogram in hypokalemia. Circulation 1960: **21,** 505.

HYPOTHERMIA

34. Emslie-Smith, D., et al.: The significance of changes in the electrocardiogram in hypothermia. Brit. Heart J. 1959: **21,** 343.

ALTERNANS

35. Kimura, E., and Yoshida, K.: A case showing electrical alternans of the T wave without change in the QRS complex. Am. Heart J. 1963: **65,** 391.
36. McGregor, M., and Baskind, E.: Electrical alternans in pericardial effusion. Circulation 1955: **11,** 837.
37. Mullican, W. S., and Fisch, C.: Postextrasystolic alternation of the U wave due to hypokalemia. Am. Heart J. 1964: **68,** 383.

CARDIOMYOPATHY

38. Braudo, M., et al.: A distinctive electrocardiogram in muscular subaortic stenosis due to septal hypertrophy. Am. J. Cardiol. 1964: **14,** 599.
39. Farrokh, A. et al.: Amyloid heart disease. Am. J. Cardiol. 1964: **13,** 750.
40. Goodwin, J. F., et al.: Obstructive cardiomyopathy simulating aortic stenosis. Brit. Heart J. 1960: **22,** 403.
41. Marriott, H. J. L.: Electrocardiographic abnormalities, conduction disorders and arrhythmias in primary myocardial disease. Prog. Cardiovasc. Dis. 1964: **7,** 99.
42. Ruttenberg, H. D., et al.: Glycogen-storage disease of the heart. Am. Heart J. 1964: **67,** 469.

INTRACRANIAL HEMORRHAGE

43. Burch, G. E., et al.: A new electrocardiographic pattern observed in cerebrovascular accidents. Circulation 1954: **9,** 719.
44. Hersch, C.: Electrocardiographic changes in subarachnoid haemorrhage, meningitis, and intracranial space-occupying lesions. Brit. Heart J. 1964: **26,** 785.
45. Surawicz, B.: Electrocardiographic pattern of cerebrovascular accident. J.A.M.A. 1966: **197,** 913.

Review Tracing

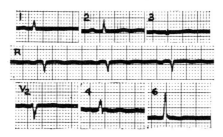

TR-39
For interpretation, see pages 314–17

Review Tracings

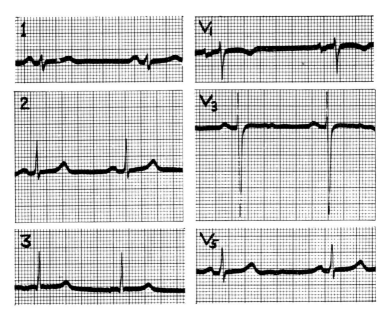

TR-40

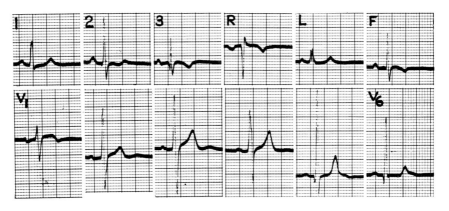

TR-41
For interpretations, see pages 314–17

Review Tracing

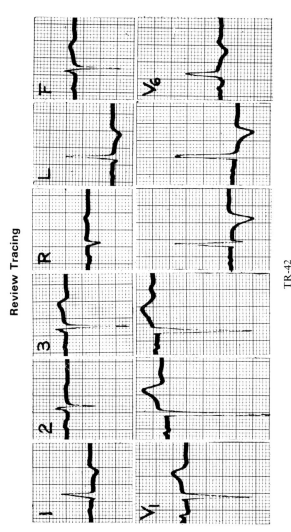

TR-42

For interpretation, see pages 314–17

Review Tracings: Interpretations

TR-1, page 126: Left ventricular hypertrophy and strain. (From a 34-year-old man with coarctation of the aorta.)

TR-2, page 126: 1) Right bundle-branch block. 2) The third beat in each lead is a ventricular premature beat. 3) Thanks to the respite of the long compensatory pause, the beat following the extrasystole is conducted with less block—incomplete RBBB—a manifestation of "critical rate."

TR-3, page 127: Ventricular tachycardia. Note charactristic features: qR with early peak in V_1, QS in V_6 and bizarre frontal plane axis ($-135°$).

TR-4, page 151: Right ventricular hypertrophy and strain with right atrial hypertrophy as well. From a patient with pulmonic stenosis and tricuspid insufficiency resulting from the malignant carcinoid syndrome.

TR-5, page 151: 1) The second beat is a supraventricular premature beat. 2) The fourth beat is a ventricular premature beat.

TR-6, page 152: 1) Atrial fibrillation. 2) Two ectopic ventricular beats. 3) Left ventricular hypertrophy and strain. From a patient with rheumatic heart disease with mitral and aortic involvement.

At times (beginning of lead 2, end of lead aVF) atrial activity is regular enough to be called flutter; so rhythm might be called flutter-fibrillation.

TR-7, page 166: 1) Atrial fibrillation. 2) Right bundle-branch block with 3) primary T-wave changes (to which digitalis might be contributing). 4) Marked left axis deviation (about $-90°$) presumably due to left anterior hemiblock.

TR-8, page 166: 1) Atrial flutter with varying A-V block (atrial rate about 330, ventricular about 102). 2) Right bundle-branch block, incomplete.

TR-9, page 167: A-V nodal tachycardia. (It is impossible to be certain whether the inverted P' waves seen immediately after the QRS complex are retrograde P waves from the A-V node representing "lower" nodal tachycardia, or if they are ectopic atrial waves conducted to the *following* QRS with prolonged P'R interval of about 0.40 sec. It would therefore be better to call the rhythm supraventricular tachycardia.) Sinus rhythm is restored in the bottom strip.

TR-10, page 183: Shifting (wandering) pacemaker with numerous atrial fusion beats.

TR-11, page 183: 1) Intra-atrial block. 2) First degree A-V block (P-R interval 0.22 to 0.24 sec.). 3) Shifting atrial pacemaker. 4) Numerous atrial premature beats, in V_1 producing bigeminy. The third atrial premature beat in V₁ shows 5) aberrant ventricular conduction of RBBB type. 6) Left ventricular hypertrophy and strain (judging by the high voltage of the QRS and the ST-T pattern).

TR-12, page 184: 1) Atrial fibrillation. 2) Left bundle-branch block.

TR-13, page 192: 1) Atrial premature beats. 2) Varying patterns of aberrant ventricular conduction of the premature beats.

TR-14, page 192: 1) Sinus tachycardia. 2) Wolff-Parkinson-White syndrome, type A.

TR-15, page 193: 1) Atrial fibrillation with rapid ventricular response. 2) Ventricular aberration of RBBB type.

TR-16, page 209: Second degree A-V block with Wenckebach periods—the dropped beat occurs after three conducted beats at beginning of top strip and at end of bottom strip.

TR-17, page 210: 1) Wolff-Parkinson-White syndrome, type B.

TR-18, page 210: 1) Type I second degree A-V block, including 3:2 Wenckebach periods and 2:1 block. 2) RBBB. (Note: The "A-V" block could, in fact, be due to simultaneous LBBB—see page 83.)

TR-19, page 218: 1) Intra-atrial block (P-mitrale). 2) Shifting atrial pacemaker. 3) Ventricular extrasystoles with retrograde conduction to atria. 4) Nodal escape beats terminate the compensatory pauses following the extrasystoles. From a patient with severe mitral stenosis.

TR-20, page 218: 1) Sinus arrhythmia. 2) Accelerated idionodal rhythm at rate 90 resulting in intermittent isorhythmic A-V dissociation.

TR-21, page 218: 1) Second degree A-V block with Wenckebach period. 2) A-V nodal escape beats. (From an asymptomatic 6-year-old girl.)

TR-22, page 219: 1) P waves are inverted in 2, 3 and aVF, upright in aVR; this is therefore an ectopic atrial (? coronary sinus) rhythm. 2) 2:1 A-V block (atrial rate 84, ventricular 42) with prolonged P-R in conducted beats. 3) Left ventricular hypertrophy and strain. 4) Digitalis effect.

TR-23, page 225: 1) Abnormal non-specific ST-T pattern. 2) The third beat in each lead is a premature ventricular beat. 3) Following the premature beats retrograde conduction to the atria occurs (retrograde P waves are seen deforming the ST segments). 4) Post-extrasystolic T wave changes (increase in depth of T-wave inversion) are noted in the cycles following the premature beats. From a patient with severe hypertension.

TR-24, page 225: 1) Artificial pacemaker, partially ineffective, pacing right ventricle. 2) Right ventricular escape beats.

TR-25, page 225: Ventricular beats are grouped in pairs because of the following sequence: P wave 1 is conducted to the ventricles with a P-R of 0.21 (first degree A-V block); P wave 2 is blocked and the impulse fails to activate the ventricles (second degree A-V block); P wave 3 might have been conducted but it was anticipated by a nodal escape beat. This sequence is then repeated.

TR-26, page 250: Acute extensive anterior myocardial infarction.

TR-27, page 250: 1) First degree A-V block (P-R = about 0.34 sec.). 2) Acute inferior infarction.

TR-28, page 251: Atypical intermittent left intraventricular block. Precordial leads show classical LBBB, but the block is not typical since there is a prominent Q wave in lead 1, which strongly suggests anteroseptal infarction. In aVR the block changes to an unblocked pattern that persists through aVL and aVF.

TR-29, page 252: 1) Right-bundle branch block. 2) Anteroseptal infarction. 3) Marked left axis deviation, presumably due to left anterior hemiblock.

TR-30, page 253: 1) Atrial fibrillation. 2) High grade A-V block; ventricular rhythm is completely regular (except for two beats referred to under 3) below) at rate 32—idionodal rhythm. 3) The fourth beat in V_3 and the third in V_5 have a somewhat different form from the dominant beats in their respective leads, have a shorter QRS interval and are slightly earlier than the next expected idioventricular beat; these then are presumably conducted supraventricular beats arising in the fibrillating atria. 4) Acute inferior infarction.

TR-31, page 265: 1) Acute anterior infarction. 2) RBBB. 3) Left anterior hemiblock.

TR-32, page 266: 1) A-V nodal rhythm. No P waves are visible preceding the QRS complexes; tiny notches are apparent at the very beginning of the ST segments in several of the leads—these are presumably retrograde P waves. 2) Acute inferior infarction.

TR-33, page 266: 1) Right bundle-branch block. 2) Inferior myocardial infarction.

TR-34, page 267: 1) Atrial fibrillation. 2) Complete A-V block with idioventricular rhythm at rate about 38. 3) Multiform ventricular premature beats. This combination suggests digitalis intoxication.

TR-35, page 281: 1) A-V nodal rhythm ("lower"). 2) Incomplete RBBB. 3) Acute inferior infarction.

TR-36, page 282: 1) P-congenitale (right atrial hypertrophy). 2) Right ventricular hypertrophy and strain. Axis −165°. From a patient with pulmonic stenosis.

TR-37, page 282: Early acute lateral infarction (early ST elevation in leads 1, aVL, V6 with reciprocal changes in 3, AVF, V_{1-3}).

TR-38, page 283: 1) Right bundle-branch block (with marked right axis deviation of about +120° presumably due to left posterior hemiblock). 2) Digitalis effect.

TR-39, page 311: Low voltage of QRS with flattened T waves, without much ST displacement. A non-specific pattern but most suspicious of hypothyroidism. From a patient with severe myxedema.

TR-40, page 312: 1) Sinus bradycardia with arrhythmia, rate 43 to 55. 2) Intra-atrial block (P wave duration = 0.14 sec.) with P-mitrale; note horizontal axis of P waves ($+20°$) with vertical axis of QRS ($+90°$)—this combination is highly suggestive of mitral stenosis. From a patient with rheumatic heart disease.

TR-41, page 312: Abnormal nonspecific tracing because of ST-T abnormalities and inverted U waves (V_{5-6}). (From a 22-year-old man with rheumatic aortic and mitral insufficiency.)

TR-42, page 313: 1) Left ventricular hypertrophy and strain. 2) Intra-atrial block (presumable evidence of left atrial enlargement). 3) The left axis deviation ($-40°$) indicates the likelihood of left ventricular disease besides hypertrophy and incomplete left anterior hemiblock is a possibility.

General Index

NOTE: All initial entries are nouns. Boldface page numbers refer to primary discussions of the topics.